NATURAL HOMEMADE SKIN CARE

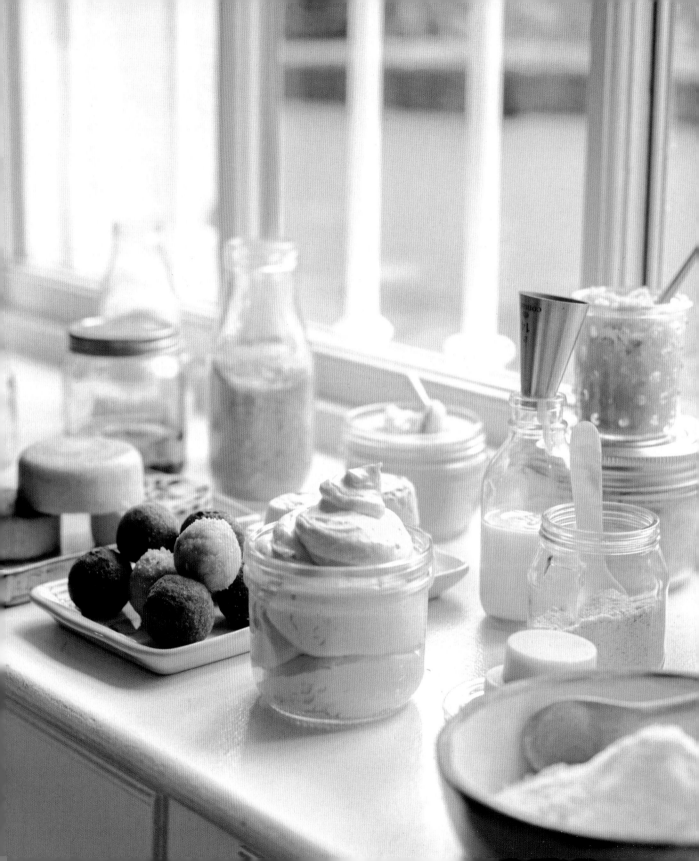

60 Cleansers, Toners,
Moisturizers and More Made
from Whole Food Ingredients

NATURAL
HOMEMADE
SKIN CARE

MILITZA MAURY

Creator of Little Green Dot

PAGE STREET
PUBLISHING CO.

PAGE STREET
PUBLISHING CO.

First published in 2020 by

Page Street Publishing Co.

27 Congress Street, Suite 105

Salem, MA 01970

www.pagestreetpublishing.com

Distributed by Macmillan, sales in Canada by The Canadian Manda Group.

24   23   22   3 4 5

ISBN-13: 978-1-64567-038-4

ISBN-10: 1-64567-038-4

Library of Congress Control Number: 2019951562

Cover and book design by Molly Gillespie for Page Street Publishing Co.

Photography by Militza Maury

Printed and bound in China

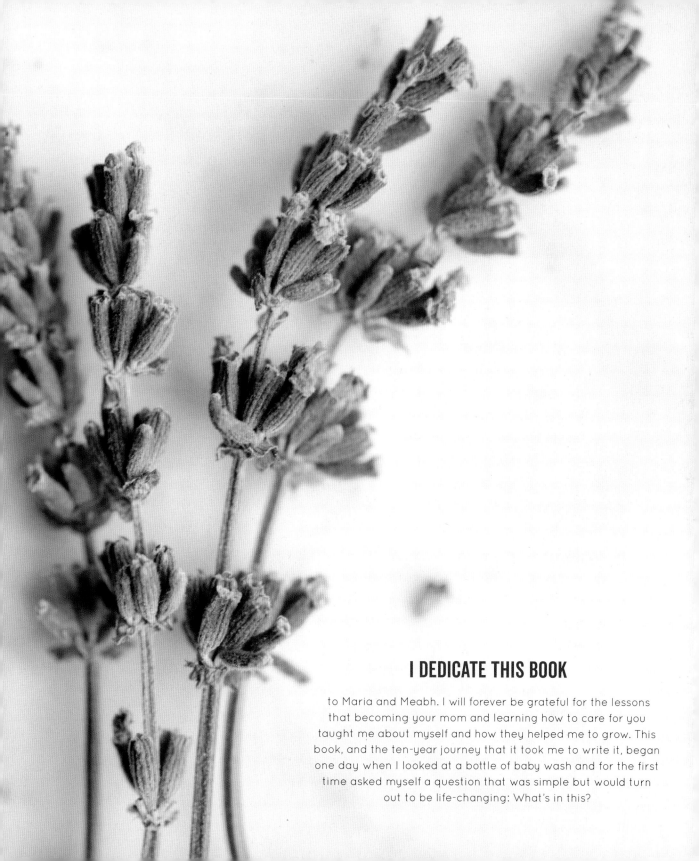

I DEDICATE THIS BOOK

to Maria and Meabh. I will forever be grateful for the lessons
that becoming your mom and learning how to care for you
taught me about myself and how they helped me to grow. This
book, and the ten-year journey that it took me to write it, began
one day when I looked at a bottle of baby wash and for the first
time asked myself a question that was simple but would turn
out to be life-changing: What's in this?

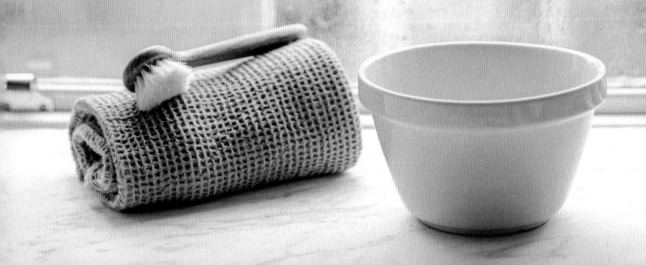

CONTENTS

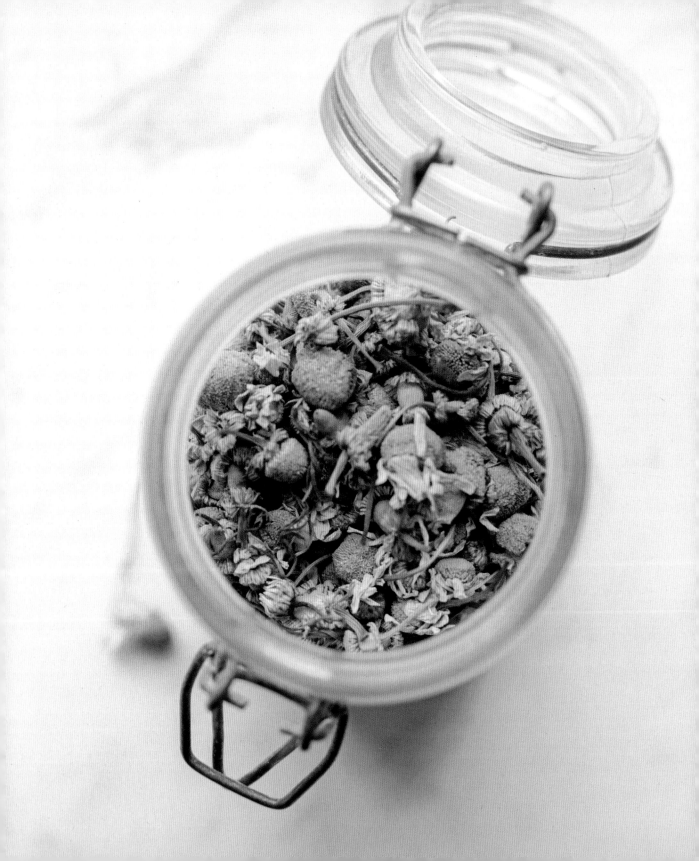

Introduction

I still remember the first skin-care recipe I ever made. It was that transformative!

I was a new mom when I discovered that the brand of baby care products I'd been using on my daughter contained potentially toxic ingredients. I ran to the nearest health-food store looking for an organic alternative but, checking the price tag, realized this was never going to be an affordable option for me. I remember how frustrated I felt. I was being forced to compromise between the health of my family and breaking the bank.

But, as I looked at the packaging of the baby bath wash in my hand, it hit me. "Made with real oats, lavender, chamomile and cocoa butter." This was basically a recipe! I could make this! I put the bath wash down and left the health-food store with an armful of ingredients instead.

Later, in my kitchen, I had no idea what I was doing. I just did what came naturally and made my daughter's skin care the same way I prepared her food: from scratch. But that night, the moment my homemade Bath Tea (page 134) slipped into my baby's bathwater, I could smell the aroma of chamomile and cocoa butter on my baby's skin—so delicate and pure—and I was hooked!

My first experiences formed my philosophy on skin care. Making skin-care products should be simple and practical, so it can become a part of your lifestyle. The ingredients should be readily available, found in the grocery store or health-food store. And it should be affordable, so that everyone can access safe and natural skin care.

This book is your complete guide to creating exquisite natural skin care that rivals anything you'll find in a store. To help make natural skin care an everyday habit for you, I'll show you how to create a simple routine you'll love (see Crafting a Routine on page 13). Over time, you'll make recipes to replace nearly all of your store-bought skin-care products: cleansers, toners, moisturizers and more.

Every recipe in this book is designed to be practical and effective. Most of the recipes are self-preserving, so you won't need to store (and forget!) your products in the refrigerator. Instead, your Sunrise Body Oil (page 76) will be ready to go, so that when you start the day you can wake up all of your senses. Your Creamy Cleansing Balm (page 26) will be right on your bathroom counter, so that you can apply it every day and see the results.

The ingredients in this book—whole foods, plant oils, herbs and butters—are carefully chosen so they can be found in your local supermarket or health-food store. You'll be amazed at the variety of skin-care products you can make from the same simple ingredients. And you won't break the bank on exotic specialty items that end up forgotten in the back of a cupboard. If the ingredients aren't easily found in your local shops, I've provided online resources at the back of the book (see Information about Ingredients on pages 147–148), and I've sprinkled alternatives throughout the recipes so you can adjust as you like. One of my favorite techniques to teach is how to make your own ingredients at home, so in the Information about Ingredients section, you'll find details on how to make your own herbal powders, fruit powders and orange-peel powder. These ingredients are what create fragrant, nutrient-dense and effective skin-care products.

My natural skin-care journey has taken me all over the world, from Singapore to Bali, and now back home to the United States. But my journey started with making that first recipe in my kitchen, which gave me such a sense of empowerment and joy! I hope this book inspires you to make your first recipe or to continue your own skin-care journey. I know the positive changes that come from using something you made yourself will lead you somewhere special.

Militza Maury

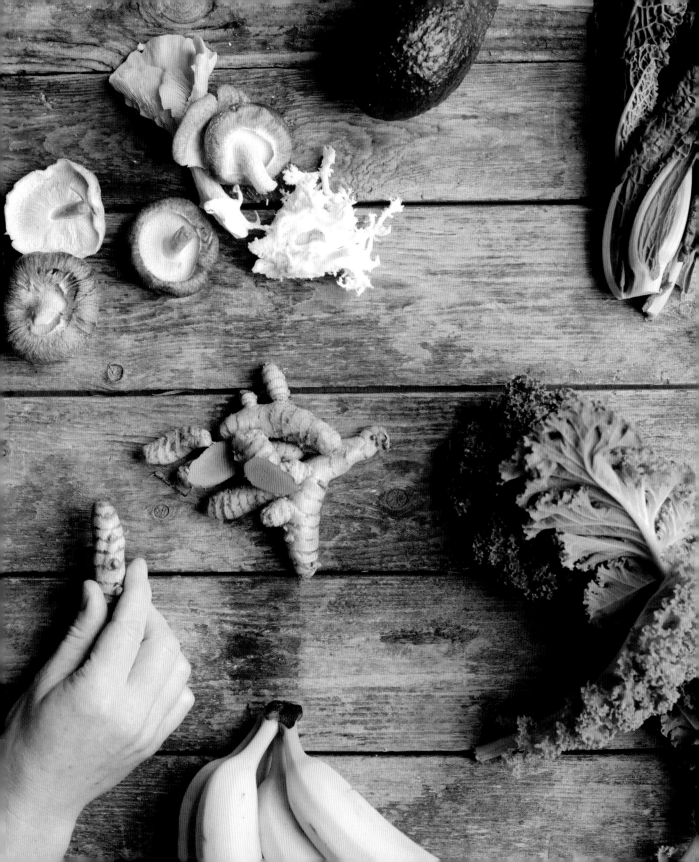

Whole Food Skin Care

We know that to have a healthy body, we need a healthy lifestyle. But when it comes to our skin, we're taught that to have healthy skin, we need a product. There's a big disconnect here.

In fact, many of the skin concerns that people see—breakouts, oil imbalance, inflammation and sensitivity—come from using too many skin-care products, with too many harsh ingredients.

Fillers, fragrances and strong preservatives disrupt the skin barrier, break down the acid mantle and impede the skin's natural functions. I call this junk food skin care. It might smell and feel good in the moment, but it provides no real nourishment.

Despite what many brands claim, skin care does not heal or fix the skin. The body does that. The point of skin care is to provide the body with the care and nutrients that it needs, so that it can perform optimally. I call this whole food skin care.

At the end of the day, we use skin care because we want to see specific results. We want to look in the mirror and see a vibrant, healthy reflection. We want to feel good in our skin. But what excites me about whole food skin care is that it does all that and more.

Skin care is actually an incredible wellness tool! Your skin is a bridge between the outside world and what's going on inside your body. If making skin-care products is a way to nourish your skin, then using skin-care products is a way to communicate directly with this incredible organ—and all the ways it impacts your whole self.

The skin is an organ: I have to start here because we often forget that the skin is not separate from our body. Like all the other organs, tissues and cells in your body, your skin requires nutrients for optimal health.

It can't thrive on a diet of junk food skin care. The recipes in this book are packed with nourishment, providing the phytonutrients and fatty acids that the skin needs.

The skin is an organ of communication: The skin informs you about your inner world, the parts of yourself that you can't see. It tells you about your digestion, your liver, your circulation. Your skin tells you when you need more sleep or more water. Each and every day, your skin-care routine is an opportunity to check in with yourself, connect with your skin and learn what it's communicating.

The skin is an immune organ: The skin is an active part of our whole immune system, lined with specialized cells that respond to stress and prevent pathogens from entering the body and causing trouble. Your daily skin-care routine can play a big role in supporting a strong and healthy immune system. The recipes in this book are filled with antioxidant-rich ingredients, nourishing oils and antimicrobial herbs that reinforce the skin barrier and support those important immune functions to keep you healthy.

The skin is connected to the nervous system: Your skin is lined with millions of receptors that link directly to the brain through the nervous system. With the touch of your own hand, you can activate the parasympathetic nervous system to reassure your body and put yourself into a relaxed state for rest and repair. The recipes in this book include herbs that can help to support, strengthen and tonify the nervous system.

The skin is a sense organ: It feels good to work with the skin. Through touch alone, you can send waves of relaxation, pleasure or comfort . . . and positively change the way you feel. The magic of skin care is that it's a total sensory experience—the scent, the texture and the colors can fully engage us and bring us into the moment.

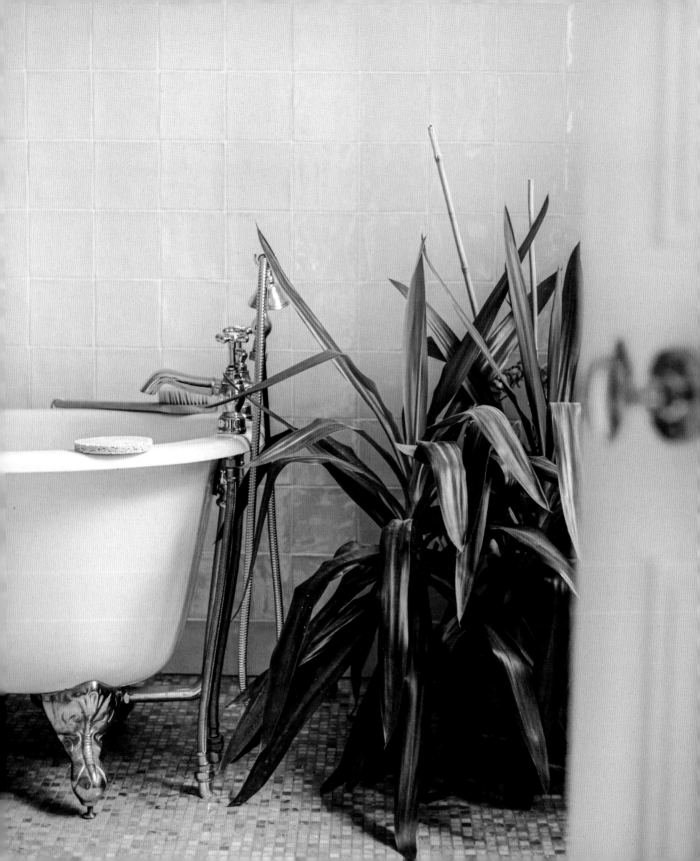

Crafting a Routine

As you begin your natural skin-care journey, it can be exciting flipping through the pages of recipes but also a little confusing knowing where exactly to start. The recipes in this book are divided by skin-care categories. The first three chapters include the steps that make up a daily skin-care routine: cleansers, toners and moisturizers. This is what you use daily to create and maintain healthy skin. Cleansers are always the first step of a routine, removing makeup, excess oils and debris. Toners are often skipped, but using a toner actually helps your skin care work more effectively. As your skin soaks in the toner, this draws nutrients deeper into your skin. So when your skin is damp with the toner, that's when you apply your moisturizer, full of nourishing oils and ingredients to feed your skin deeply!

Next, the book goes into your weekly routine: masks, scrubs and treats. This is what you'll use once or twice a week, to deeply nourish yourself.

A great place to start is with your daily routine. Choose one cleanser, one toner and one moisturizer to make—and then use them together as your full skin-care routine, every day, for two weeks. And then you can start to look at other recipes to add to your routine—a mask, a scrub and a fun treat!

When I work with clients, I always start them on what I call my Fresh-Start Routine. And I recommend it for you, too. It's a very simple daily routine, focused on helping to reset and rebalance your skin.

Fresh-Start Routine:

Cleanser: Morning: Honey Wash (page 21); Night: Makeup Melt Cleansing Oil (page 17)

Toner: Apple Cider Vinegar Toner (page 51)

Moisturizer: Makeup Melt Cleansing Oil (page 17; as the moisturizer!)

The ingredients that make up this routine are essentially honey, oil and apple cider vinegar! One trip to your health-food store, and you'll be on your way to making your skin care. And if you find yourself thinking, *This sounds almost too simple to work,* I get it! But when it comes to the skin, simple is powerful. One of my clients was in her late twenties and experiencing adult acne. When she came to me, she was feeling insecure about her skin and frustrated because she kept buying expensive products, yet saw no results!

I recommended the Fresh-Start Routine, which surprised her! She had been spending a small fortune on skin-care products, and the idea of using oil and honey sounded too simple to be effective. But she followed the routine exactly. And within the first week, she noticed results! On our call, she said "It's almost miraculous; my acne is clearing! People are complimenting my skin!"

She told me that she was going to sell her collection of branded products to her friends and that she was excited to be on this new skin-care journey.

And I can't wait for you to start, too!

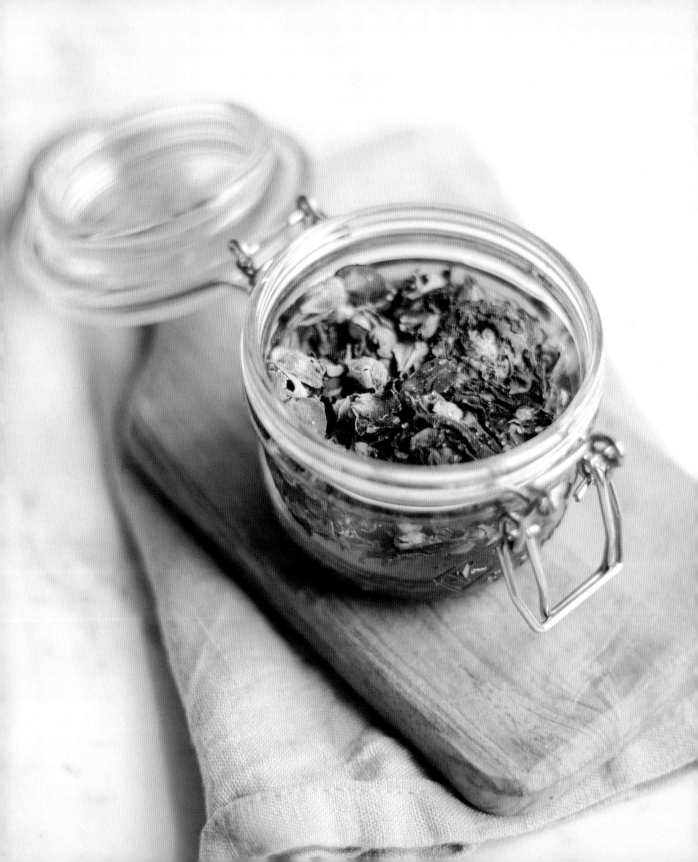

Cleansers

Have you ever washed your face with a soap cleanser and felt a dry and tight sensation afterward? Sometimes you can even feel a tingling, and that might feel like a good thing, like it's working! But is that true?

Many of the soap products on the market are simply too harsh for what the skin needs, and that squeaky-clean feeling is actually damaging the skin's natural functions, throwing everything off balance.

That's why when people come to my workshops frustrated by their skin imbalances, the first question I ask is: What cleanser are you using? I always suggest removing any synthetically made soaps and cleansers from their skin-care routine.

In this chapter, I'll show you the options that you have to clean your skin, without that drying, stripping sensation. You'll love the single-ingredient recipes, which you can probably make right now from ingredients already in your kitchen. For example, to take off your makeup, try the Makeup Melt Cleansing Oil (page 17)! It cleans your skin gently yet effectively and even removes waterproof mascara. And the Honey Wash (page 21) clears pimple-causing bacteria away—it's so good at clearing up acne and breakouts.

Then, when you're ready, you can try infusing your own oils (Herbal-Infused Oil 101 on pages 18–19) and honey (Herbal-Infused Honey 101 on page 22) to amp up the cleansing and nourishing benefits. I love hosting friends to make infusions together—everyone can bring a different herb to share!

For more skin-care making, the Deep Cleansing Powder (page 29) is one of my favorite cleansers; it gently buffs your skin clean. And the Creamy Cleansing Balm (page 26) feels so soft and gratifying on the skin—you'll love it!

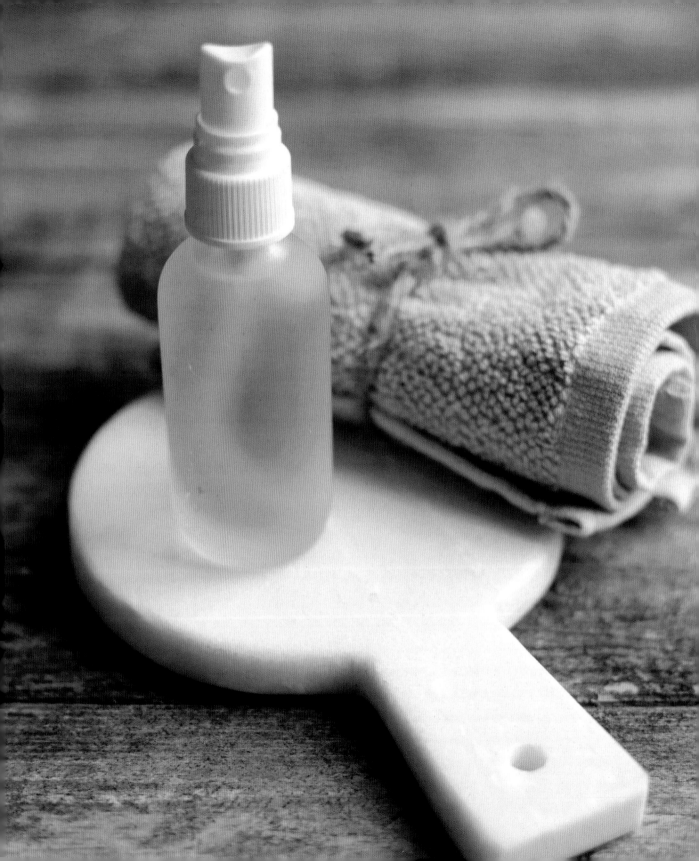

Makeup Melt Cleansing Oil

When I teach this recipe in my workshops, I feel guilty that it's almost too simple. Yet I always teach it—because this cleanser continues to be one of the most transformative for people. I suspect it works mainly because it gives the skin a break from harsh conventional cleansers. But it also works because of the oil. Jojoba oil, in my experience, is the perfect oil cleanser. It's very compatible with skin, dissolves congestion in pores and balances oil production. Massaging with jojoba oil lifts up excess oils, dirt, bacteria, makeup, pollution and impurities—and leaves your skin clean and clear. It's also gentle enough to be used around the eyes, fully removing any trace of mascara—even waterproof!

So as simple as this recipe may seem, I had to include it here, because if you've been frustrated with your skin, this may become your new favorite "recipe" to make!

Skin type: all skin types | **Shelf life:** 3–6 months

---

4 tbsp (60 ml) jojoba oil

10 drops essential oil, optional (tea tree or lavender are good choices for their cleansing effects)

TIP: You don't need to oil cleanse morning and night. I suggest that you use this oil cleanser in the evenings only, to remove makeup and buildup from the day. In the morning, freshen your skin with a cotton pad soaked in your favorite toner. I love the Chamomile Ice (page 59) to totally wake up and de-puff skin!

Purchase or repurpose a 2-ounce (60-ml) glass spray bottle. You can use any bottle—such as one with a pump top, dropper top or pour top—but I find that spraying out the oil makes it much easier to use. It's my little trick!

Sterilize the bottle with boiling water and rubbing alcohol, dry it fully and then fill it up with jojoba oil. If you are using essential oils, add the ten drops, then shake to distribute. Label your bottle.

To cleanse your skin, start with dry skin, even if you have makeup on—all the makeup will be coming off with this one cleanser. Spray four to five pumps of oil into your palms—about a half to a full teaspoon worth—and then massage the oil onto your face. Spend time on areas that are congested with blackheads, massage away tension around your jaw and temples and gently work over your eyes to remove any makeup.

After you cleanse, follow with a spray of one of the hydrosol recipes in this book (pages 40–48) or with Apple Cider Vinegar Toner (page 51). I like to spray my toner onto a cotton pad and swipe the skin as a "second" cleanser. With your skin still slightly damp from the toner, apply two to three drops of one of the two serum recipes in this book (pages 71 and 72), gently patting the oil into your skin. This three-step routine is incredibly simple, but for so many people I've worked with, it has been transformative.

Herbal-Infused Oil 101

Herbal oils are an age-old, traditional remedy, yet underrated given the benefits they can bring to our modern life. Massaging your body with oils infused with beneficial herbs not only moisturizes and nourishes skin on the surface but brings full-body wellness deep within, stimulating circulation and boosting the body's functions.

This recipe is a guide on how to infuse oil. Herb choices and exact measurements really depend on the purpose of the oil and the amount that you want to make. I always teach the "folk" or "simpler" method where you eyeball the amounts in any size jar, but the general rule of thumb is 1 ounce (28 g) of herbs to 10 ounces (295 ml) of oil.

When choosing your herbs, think about the results you want from the final product. Choose anti-inflammatory herbs to help the body better respond to stress, antibacterial herbs to cleanse and protect, vulnerary herbs to heal and mend, stimulating herbs to boost the body's functions or nutrient-rich herbs to support all the systems of the body. Aromatic herbs can also be added to a blend to bring emotional wellness: calming the nervous system, promoting sleep or uplifting the mood.

You can infuse a single herb or combine several herbs. I think keeping it simple is always best, using one to four herbs in an infusion, so that you get the most potent amount of each.

Skin type: all skin types | ***Shelf life:*** 3–6 months

---

1 cup (28 g) dried herb of choice (use a single herb or a combination of 1–4 herbs)

1¼ cups (295 ml) jojoba oil, or a neutral oil like grapeseed oil

Sterilize a 10-ounce (295-ml) Mason jar. Fill the jar one-half to three-quarters of the way full with the dried herbs, then top the herbs with oil, covering them fully and filling the jar to the rim. Label the jar with the ingredients and the date you made the infusion. There are two ways to infuse the oil. Cold infusions take more time but require no work. Warm infusions require a few more steps and equipment but are ready much sooner. Warm infusion is my preferred method because it takes 6 hours versus 6 weeks!

Cold infusion: Set the jar in a cupboard and let it infuse for 4 to 6 weeks. Every day, visit the jar and shake the contents to encourage the infusion.

Warm infusion: The important thing with heating oils is that you need a controlled and precise heat setting: 110°F (40°C). If you have an oven that can be set as low as 110°F (40°C), put the lid on the jar and place it in the oven over a tray. Leave the jar in the oven for 6 hours (or longer, for more potency). Alternatively, you can use a sous vide machine. With a sous vide, you can set the temperature to exactly 110°F (40°C) and place several jars of various oils inside to infuse. Many herbalists love the MagicalButter machine, which has a low setting control and periodically stirs the oils. Slow cookers can get too hot, and it is hard to control the temperature on the stovetop. We don't want to overheat the oils and degrade the medicinal properties.

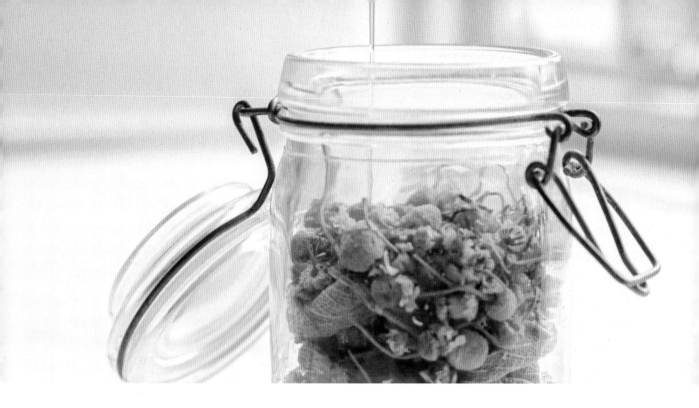

Six hours of infusing under heat will extract a lot of aromatic and herbal benefits. But the longer you infuse the oil, the stronger it becomes. Many herbalists will infuse oils throughout the whole day, or for as many as 10 days! If you have the patience, I recommend giving it extra time. You will make a skin-care product that is so potent and healing!

When the oil has been infused, whether by the cold or warm method, strain out the herbs. Use a fine-mesh strainer lined with a cheesecloth to make sure you do not get pieces of herbs in your final product.

To use your herbal oil, apply it directly onto your skin, as a moisturizer. You can use herbal oil on your face, body and hair. Add herbal oil to a bath or foot bath. And you can use your herbal oil in any of the recipes that call for "oil."

TIP: My favorite healthy-skin blend includes:

Sage: antibacterial, antifungal and astringent actions, toning tissue. Sage is also an aromatic, uplifting a dull mood.

Chamomile: anti-inflammatory actions, soothing stress and building resilience. Chamomile is also an aromatic that calms feelings of stress and anxiety.

Calendula: vulnerary (skin healing) and lymphatic actions, draining excess fluid and toxins.

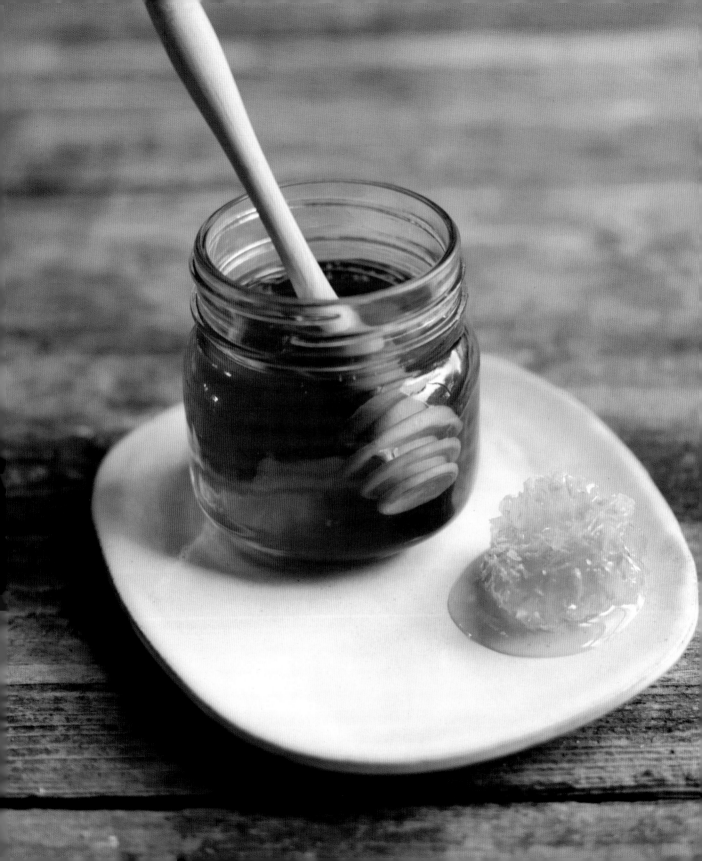

Honey Wash

I once created a challenge for my blog readers: See what happens if you stop using conventional cleansers for one week and instead, wash your skin with honey. Thousands of people signed up, and the results were incredible! Emails poured in from people who saw their skin transform and even had acne clear up, simply by replacing their cleanser with one simple ingredient! Honey is enzyme rich; stimulates cell production and collagen production; is healing, antibacterial and anti-inflammatory; lightens dark spots; and hydrates the deep layers of skin. Honey is as simple as it gets with making your own skin care, but when it's this effective, what more do you need?

Skin type: all skin types; especially good for acne-prone skin | **Shelf life:** 3 months

---

1 tbsp (15 ml) raw, unfiltered honey

To use, first remove your makeup with the Makeup Melt Cleansing Oil (page 17). After removing your makeup, lightly dampen your skin with water or a spritz of hydrosol (pages 40–48), so that the honey applies easily. Don't wet your skin too much, or the honey will dissolve! Apply a generous tablespoon (15 ml) of honey onto your face and neck, and let it sit for 15 minutes to allow the cleansing action of the honey to work on your skin. Then wash off the honey with water. I prefer to apply the honey right before a shower because it is easier to remove the honey under the stream of water in the shower.

Use the Honey Wash daily to keep your skin healthy and hydrated.

TIPS: Source your honey from your local farmers' market where you can speak to the person behind the product or purchase a reputable brand. It's so important to source honey carefully from people who work to support a healthy population of bees and that never alter the honey with chemicals or heat.

If you find honey that comes packaged in a squeeze bottle, it will be even easier to use! Simply squeeze the honey into the palm of your hands. If your honey comes in a glass jar, I recommend repurposing a squeeze bottle for storing your Honey Wash. Sometimes honey is thick and creamy, which feels amazing on the skin! If your honey is thick, keep it in the jar it came packaged in and use a clean spoon to scoop it out for each use.

Herbal-Infused Honey 101

Infusing honey with herbs is a wonderful way to extract the healing properties of a plant and bring those benefits to your skin. Honey draws out water-soluble vitamins like vitamin C; astringent tannins, which tonify the skin; and the natural acids and aromatics from the herbs. The infused honey will be fragrant (and flavorful), and you can customize the herbs to suit your needs and wants. Rose honey is especially good to plump and tone skin.

When it comes to choosing herbs or a blend of herbs to infuse into honey, I suggest reading Herbal-Infused Oil 101 (pages 18–19), as many of the principles for infusing are the same here.

Skin type: all skin types | ***Shelf life:*** 3–6 months

¼ cup (9 g) dried rose petals (or 1 part herb of choice)

1 cup (240 ml) raw, unfiltered honey (or 4 parts honey)

Scoop the rose petals into a clean, sterilized jar. Pour in the honey, fully covering the rose petals. Stir well to combine, making sure there are no air bubbles and that the petals are all fully saturated in honey. I like to use chopsticks or the long handle of a spoon for mixing. Tighten the lid of the jar, and make sure to label and date the jar. Set a reminder in your calendar to strain out the honey in 2 weeks. This will produce an aromatic honey; for more potent healing actions, allow it to infuse for 4 weeks.

Every day, flip the jar so that the honey moves with the herbs, helping to release the constituents of the rose petals. When you are ready to strain, gently warm the honey in a bowl of hot water, so that it softens and pours more easily. Pour the honey through a sieve to capture the rose petals, then put the infused honey in a bottle.

To use your infused honey, follow the directions in the Honey Wash recipe (page 21).

TIPS: For calming sunburned, irritated or inflamed skin, try infusing chamomile into honey. If you have chamomile tea, just tear open a few tea bags and pour the chamomile tea leaves into the honey! Another favorite of mine is lavender honey, to use both on skin experiencing breakouts and also as a drink in the evenings (with warm milk) as a sleepy-time remedy. The beauty of herbs is that they are holistic, bringing wellness inside and out.

You can scale this recipe up or down as needed—just make sure to use 1 part herbs to 4 parts honey.

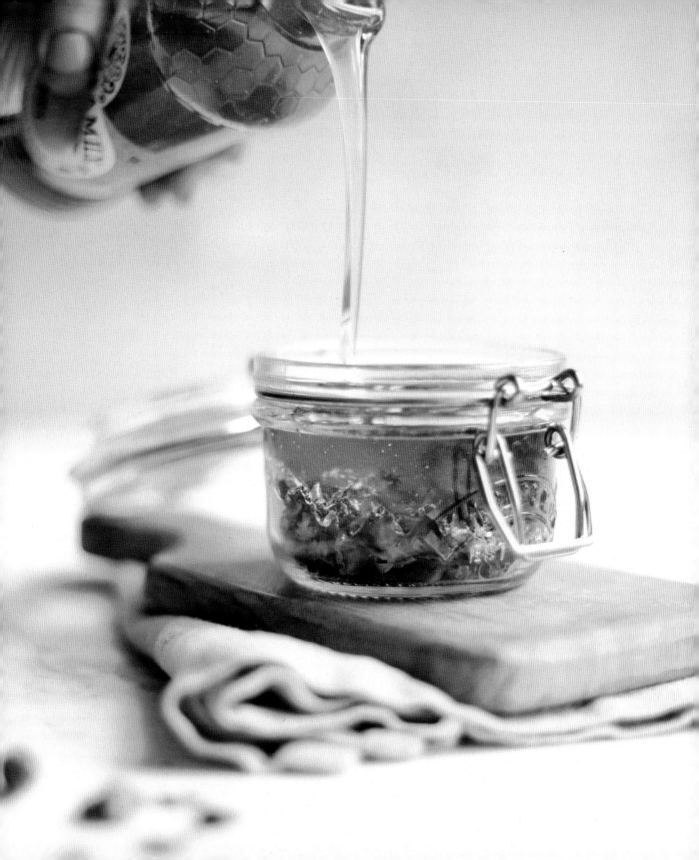

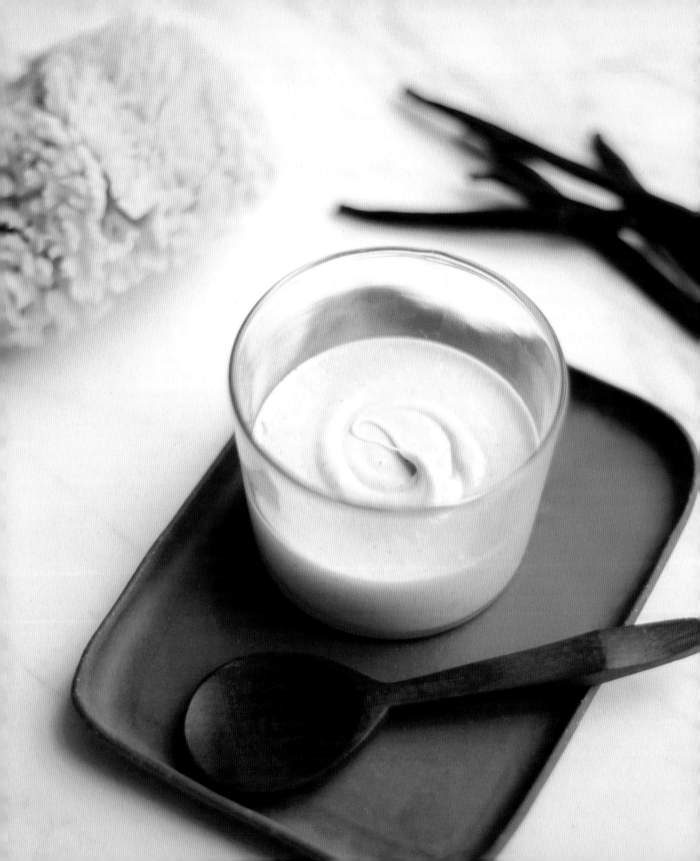

Thick Honey Cleanser

Deep cleansing and hydrating. Stimulating and soothing. Detoxifying and nourishing. This cleanser has the best of it all, with just two active ingredients: honey and clay. When my daughter's hormonal acne is triggered, this is my one-stop solution to keep her skin calm and clear. It almost instantly brings down inflammation and redness around pimples, and with daily use for one week, it helps to prevent new ones from forming. I recommend using this when you see inflammation and breakouts. But using it once per week is also a great way to deeply cleanse.

In addition to being great for breakouts, this Thick Honey Cleanser also brightens, plumps and tones the skin. In my family, it takes care of two generations of women and our different needs!

A touch of vanilla in this recipe gives antibacterial support, but mostly, it makes the product feel comforting and satisfying on the skin—to me it's like dipping into a cup of vanilla pudding!

Skin type: dull, dehydrated, congested or inflamed skin | *Shelf life:* 3 months

---

¼ cup (60 ml) raw honey

5 drops essential oil of choice (for example, lavender), optional

6 tbsp (30 g) kaolin clay

Seeds from ¼ of a vanilla pod

Pour or scoop the raw honey into a bowl. If you are using essential oils, add them to the honey and stir to combine. Add the clay, a little at a time, to the honey, and stir to combine. The consistency of honey varies, so you may need to add only a small amount of clay at a time until the mixture reaches a thick, spreadable consistency. Add the vanilla seeds and continue mixing until well combined.

To use, remove any makeup with the Makeup Melt Cleansing Oil (page 17). Lightly dampen your skin, then apply the Thick Honey Cleanser all over your face and neck. Leave the cleanser on for 10 minutes, then remove with a warm cotton cloth or in the shower under a stream of water.

Store the Thick Honey Cleanser in a widemouthed jar that you can easily scoop into. Make sure to use clean, dry fingers or a spoon with each use, so that you don't introduce bacteria or water into the product.

TIP: You can add essential oils to this recipe—you might try lavender or tea tree for acne or Roman chamomile for inflammation. Adding essential oils will alter the scent of vanilla, but you can leave out the vanilla if you wish.

Creamy Cleansing Balm

Cleansing balms feel cozy on the skin; the texture is incredibly creamy and satisfying. As a cleanser, it works in the same way as using an oil—lifting and removing dirt, makeup and bacteria from skin. But you may prefer the feel and use of a solid balm product. I do find that balms are less messy and easier to travel with than liquid oils, and I enjoy the richer feel on my skin. The addition of beeswax creates the solid consistency and also provides added healing and anti-inflammatory properties.

Skin type: all skin types | **Shelf life:** 6 months

¼ cup (56 g) beeswax

10 drops lavender essential oil

1 cup (240 ml) jojoba oil

In a double boiler, or a bowl set over a pot of simmering water, place the beeswax. While the beeswax begins to melt, add the essential oil to the jar you will be using for storing the final product. I recommend using a shallow jar with a wide mouth; this will allow you to easily scoop out the product.

When the beeswax is fully melted, add the jojoba oil. With the addition of the oil, the beeswax will congeal, but after a few seconds, it will become a liquid golden pool again. Remove the bowl from the heat, let the mixture cool for about 5 minutes before it begins to harden, and then pour the melted liquid into the jar containing the essential oil. As you pour it in, the essential oil will swirl around and incorporate into the mixture. Close the lid and let it sit in the refrigerator for 15 minutes to firm up. At that point, you can remove it from the refrigerator and keep the balm by your bathroom sink.

To use, start with dry skin (it's okay if you still have makeup on). Scoop out a small dollop of balm (roughly a teaspoon), and begin massaging it onto your face and neck. Close your eyes and enjoy the massage. You can use this cleanser over your eyes to remove eye makeup. When you are done, just as you would do with all oil-based cleansers, use a soft cotton cloth and water to remove the product from your skin, lifting up the oils that trap dirt, makeup and bacteria.

TIP: This cleanser also works as a moisturizing balm. You can use it on dry skin, on your cuticles or even on the tips of your hair.

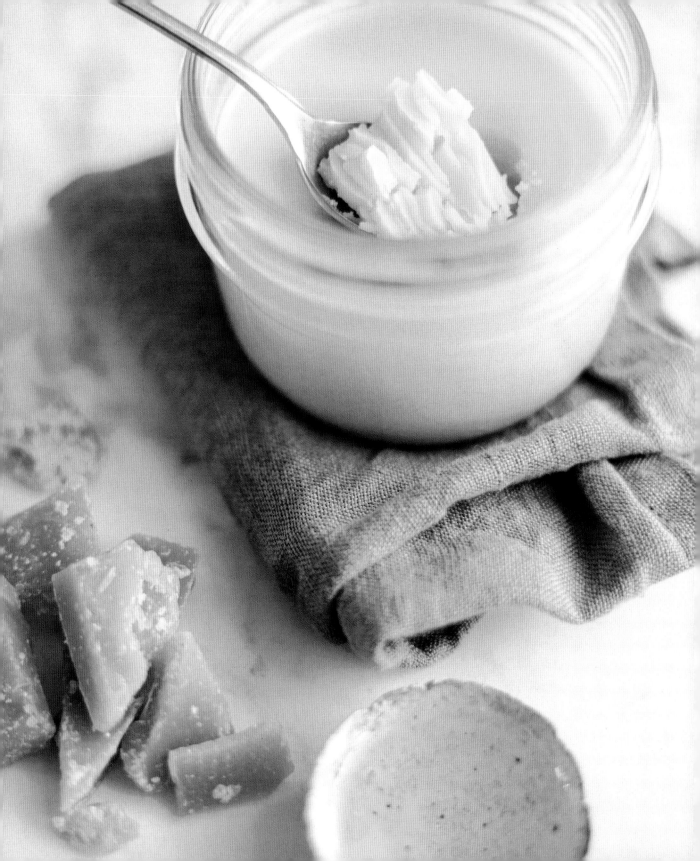

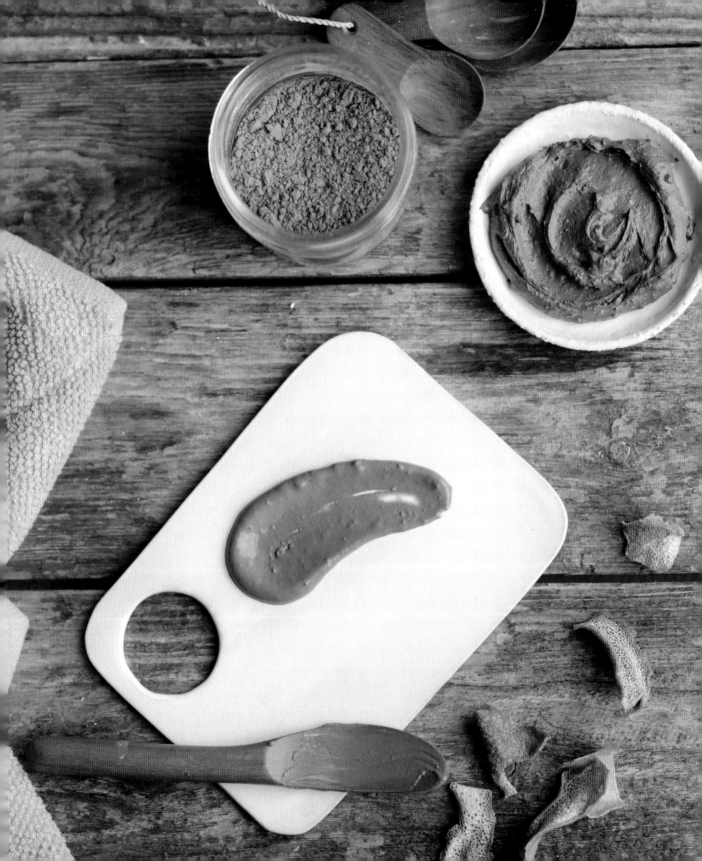

Deep Cleansing Powder

This cleansing blend starts out as a powder and becomes a creamy cleanser when mixed with water. Made with detoxifying clay and stimulating herbs, you'll feel its warmth on your skin as it encourages circulation and lymphatic drainage, brightens and evens your complexion, calms inflammation, releases congestion and prevents breakouts. This blend is especially good for waking up lackluster or dull skin, but I also recommend using it as a reset—for one week, every new season of the year—to stimulate and boost natural functions and to maintain vitality.

Skin type: all skin types, especially dull skin | ***Shelf life:*** 3-6 months

---

¼ cup (20 g) kaolin clay

¼ cup (24 g) dried calendula powder (see Information about Ingredients, pages 147-148)

¼ cup (20 g) cacao powder

1 tbsp (5 g) ginger powder

1 tbsp (5 g) orange peel powder (see Information about Ingredients, pages 147-148)

Choose a container for storing your final product—I like repurposing a glass jam jar. Make sure it's clean and completely dry.

Add the clay and the calendula, cacao, ginger and orange peel powders to the container, close the lid and shake well to incorporate.

To use, scoop out about 1 tablespoon (5 g) of the powder and add it to a small bowl. Drizzle droplets of water onto the powder and stir. Continue adding drops of water and stirring until the mixture is thick yet creamy.

First cleanse your skin with the Makeup Melt Cleansing Oil (page 17) or Creamy Cleansing Balm (page 26). Remove the product from your skin with a warm cloth. Apply the Deep Cleansing Powder to your skin and let it sit for 10 to 15 minutes, misting your skin with water or hydrosol (pages 40-48) to keep the clay from drying out. It's important to not let clay masks dry on your skin, or they will dehydrate your skin. Another option for keeping the mask moist is to leave it on for 5 to 7 minutes and, just before it dries, step into a steamy shower, waiting until the end of your shower to remove the mask under the stream of water.

TIP: You can also add ¼ cup (20 g) of this blend to a bath for a full-body treatment.

Moisturizing Milk Cleanser

This creamy, milky blend restores dry and dehydrated skin. Oat milk soothes, coconut milk moisturizes and buttermilk revitalizes skin cells. For added dewiness, I choose vitamin C-rich rose petals to boost collagen, tone the skin and help better retain hydration.

Skin type: all skin types; especially good for dry, dull and dehydrated skin |
Shelf life: 3 months

---

1 tbsp (8 g) oat powder (see Information about Ingredients, pages 147–148, or try colloidal oats for an extra creamy and smooth texture)

1 tbsp (8 g) coconut milk powder

1 tbsp (11 g) buttermilk powder

1 tbsp (4 g) rose petal powder (see Information about Ingredients, pages 147–148)

Add the oat, coconut milk, buttermilk and rose petal powders to a small jar. Seal the lid and shake to mix all the ingredients together.

To use, scoop out about a tablespoon (8 g) of the powder into a small bowl. Drizzle droplets of water onto the powder and stir. Continue slowly adding drops of water and stirring until the mixture is creamy but thin.

Apply the mixture onto clean skin, and let it sit for 15 minutes. Remove with a soft cloth and water or in the shower.

TIPS: If your skin is so dry that it's chapping, add 1 tablespoon (4 g) of dried calendula powder (see Information about Ingredients, pages 147–148) to your blend for its healing benefits. You can always customize the herbs to speak to your needs!

This formula is very simple, being one part of each ingredient, so you can scale it up easily. I recommend using this blend for one week to see how your skin responds. After the one-week test, you can decide if you want to make a larger batch next time or make any changes to the recipe.

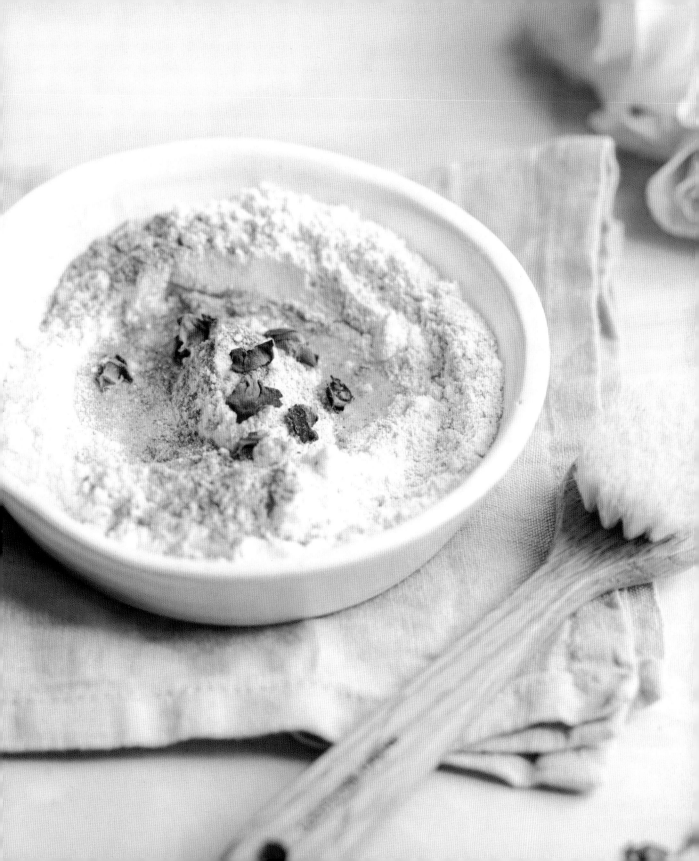

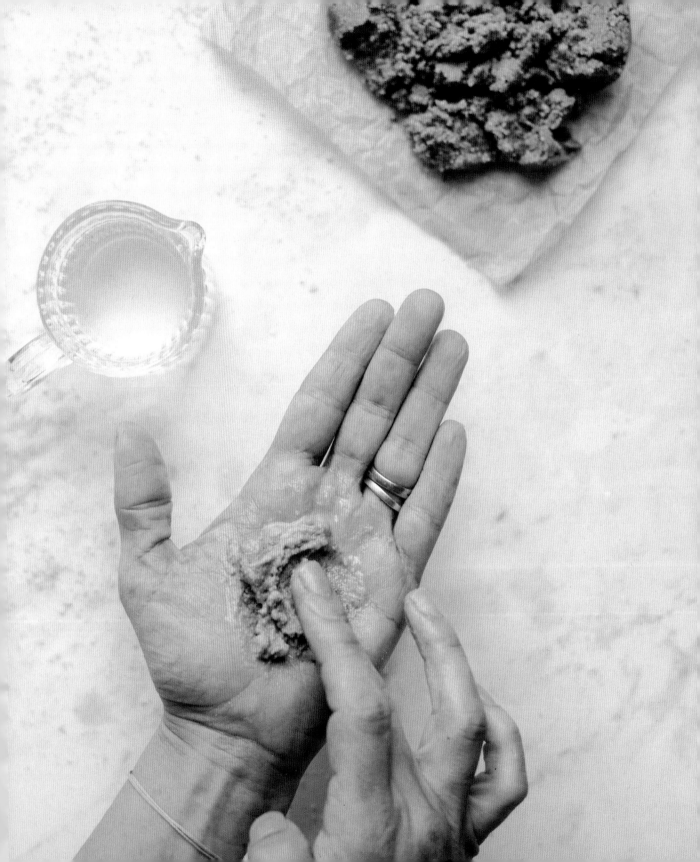

Energizing Cookie Dough Cleanser

This cleanser is dense and rich, like cookie dough in your hands! When mixed with water, the texture becomes light and creamy, the botanical elements come to life and the herbs release their healing constituents. This blend features maca, a root traditionally used to enhance vitality—it brings energy to your skin cells and helps to reduce the signs of aging.

Skin type: all skin types; especially good for dull skin | ***Shelf life:*** 1 month, or up to 3 months in the refrigerator

---

3 tbsp (24 g) almond flour

2 tbsp (24 g) maca powder (see Information about Ingredients, pages 147–148)

1 tbsp (15 ml) + ¼ tsp (if needed) jojoba oil or Facial Serum (page 71)

TIP: This cleanser travels well. Pinch off what you need and store it in a little container to take it with you.

When you're making a large amount of this cleanser it's best to make this recipe in a stand mixer with a paddle attachment. It's just like baking, and the "dough" comes together perfectly! If you don't have a stand mixer or if you're only making a small amount (and this recipe is for a small amount), use a large bowl and silicone spatula, which lets you smear and mix the ingredients well.

Combine the almond flour and maca powder in the stand-mixer bowl or a large bowl. Mix well to fully incorporate. Slowly begin to drizzle in the oil, working it through well, breaking up clumps and adding more oil gradually until it comes together to form a cookie dough–like texture. If the dough is crumbly or dry, add the extra ¼ teaspoon of jojoba oil or Facial Serum and mix until the dough comes together well.

Scrape the dough out of the bowl and onto a piece of parchment paper. Roll it up into a log shape and cut off one cookie-sized slice (about 2 to 3 tablespoons [30 to 45 g]). Keep it in an airtight container by your sink. Wrap the rest of the dough in parchment paper and store it in the refrigerator. This way you know your product is good and fresh!

To use, first remove any makeup with the Makeup Melt Cleansing Oil (page 17). Then pinch off a piece of the doughy cleanser, about one heaping teaspoon worth. Smoosh it into the palm of your hands (or a bowl if you prefer), and begin to drizzle droplets of water onto it and stir gently until it breaks down into a creamy paste. Gently massage onto your skin. For more stimulation, I recommend leaving it on for 15 minutes for the herbal actions to wake up your skin! Wash off the cleanser with a cloth and water or in the shower under the stream of water.

Soothing Cookie Dough Cleanser

This cookie dough cleanser base features soothing oats, anti-inflammatory chamomile and cleansing lavender with matcha powder for a boost of antioxidant protection. Sensitive skin will appreciate the soft and gentle creaminess as you cleanse, with herbs focusing on soothing red, irritated and inflamed skin conditions.

Skin type: all skin types, especially inflamed skin | ***Shelf life:*** 1 month, or up to 3 months in the refrigerator

---

4 tbsp (32 g) oat powder (see Information about Ingredients, pages 147–148)

1 tbsp (3 g) lavender powder (see Information about Ingredients, pages 147–148)

2 tbsp (6 g) chamomile powder (see Information about Ingredients, pages 147–148)

1 tbsp (8 g) matcha powder (see Information about Ingredients, pages 147–148)

1 tbsp (15 ml) + ¼ tsp (if needed) oil of choice (I recommend jojoba or sesame; you can also use Makeup Melt Cleansing Oil [page 17])

In a small bowl, stir together the oat, lavender, chamomile and matcha powders until well incorporated. Slowly drizzle in the oil, and with a silicone spatula, break up any clumps and combine to create a cookie dough–like texture. Add the extra ¼ teaspoon of oil if the "dough" is dry or crumbly; this should be just enough for the mixture to come together.

Store the mixture in an airtight container or wrap in parchment paper and keep it in the refrigerator. This recipe will keep outside of the refrigerator for one month, but I prefer to keep the bulk of the product refrigerated and only keep what I'll use in a week in a jar in the bathroom.

To use, remove makeup with the Makeup Melt Cleansing Oil (page 17). Then pinch off a piece of the doughy cleanser, about one heaping teaspoon worth. Smoosh it into the palm of your hands (or a bowl if you prefer), and begin to drizzle droplets of water onto it until it breaks down into a creamy paste. Massage the cleanser onto your skin. Enjoy the gentle exfoliation from the herbal powders, focusing your attention on areas that may have congested pores. Wash the cleanser off with a cloth and water or in the shower under the stream of water.

TIP: You can also use this cleanser on your neck, chest, breasts, stomach and arms.

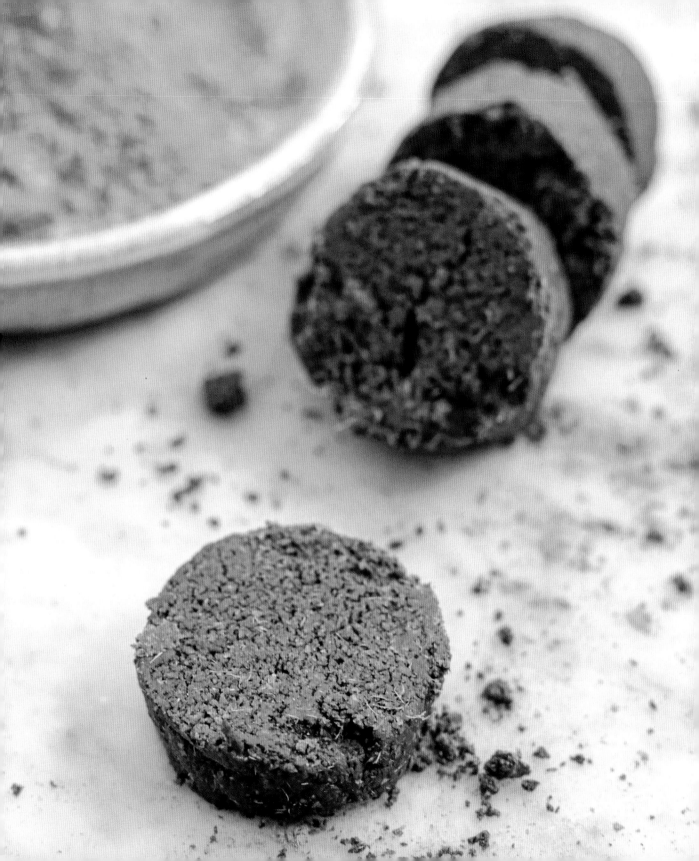

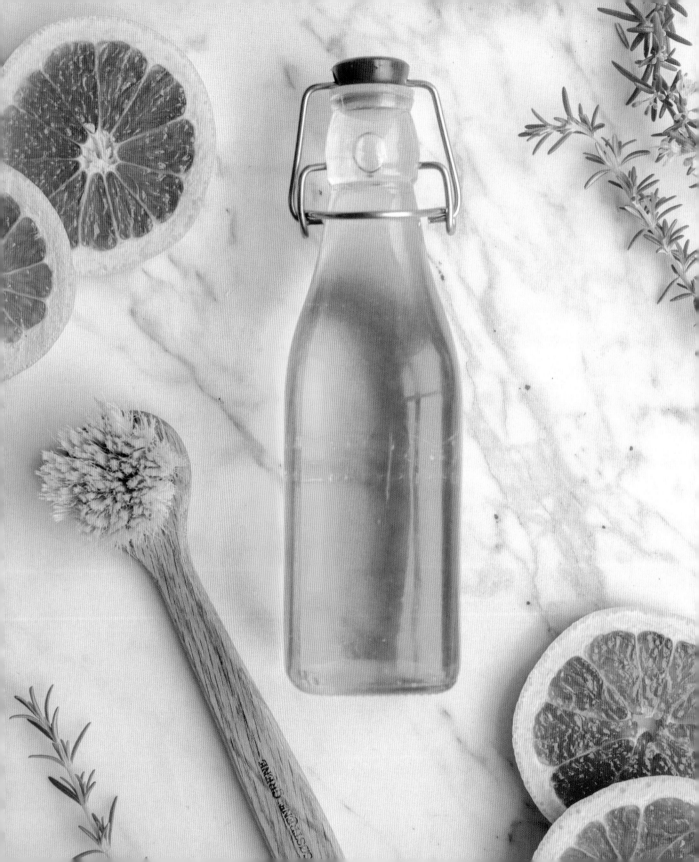

Sesame-Citrus Body-Cleansing Oil

Sesame oil is a wonderful choice for cleansing—it's antibacterial and antifungal, clearing the skin of common pathogens and fungi. It has a detoxifying effect on the body, creating warmth and circulation, which supports the clearing out of toxins and nourishes the cells. Sesame oil is a thick oil; it feels silky on your skin and relaxes the body. Massage your skin every day before you step into the shower to cleanse, stimulate and deeply nourish your entire body. In this recipe, jojoba oil tones down the nutty scent of the raw sesame oil, with a touch of aromatic grapefruit and rosemary essential oils to boost the cleansing benefits.

Skin type: all skin types | ***Shelf life:*** 3–6 months

¼ cup (60 ml) virgin sesame oil (do not use toasted sesame oil)

¼ cup (60 ml) jojoba oil

30 drops grapefruit essential oil

30 drops rosemary essential oil

Choose a bottle to store the oil blend. I recommend using a bottle that will let you pour the oil easily into the palm of your hand. You can repurpose a sauce bottle; just make sure it is clean and completely dry.

Pour the sesame and jojoba oils into the bottle, then add the essential oils. The full scent of the blend will settle in and develop within 24 to 48 hours, but you can start using the oil right away.

It looks beautiful to add a sprig of dried rosemary or a sliver of dried grapefruit peel to the bottle as a decorative touch. Just make sure that if you add botanicals, they are fully dried so as to not incorporate water into the oil.

To use, massage about a tablespoon (15 ml) of oil all over your body—arms, chest, breasts, stomach, buttocks and legs. Move your hands over your body in a circular motion, noticing areas that are holding tension so you can give a little more attention to those spots. The rubbing motion activates the circulation and lymph systems in the body.

This blend is formulated for the body only; I would not recommend it for the face, as it may be too stimulating. If you want to use this product head-to-toe, cut the essential oils down to a total of 20 to 30 drops.

TIP: This blend is euphoric and invigorating. It wakes up your body and senses, so use it in the morning for a boost of energy and to promote a good mood.

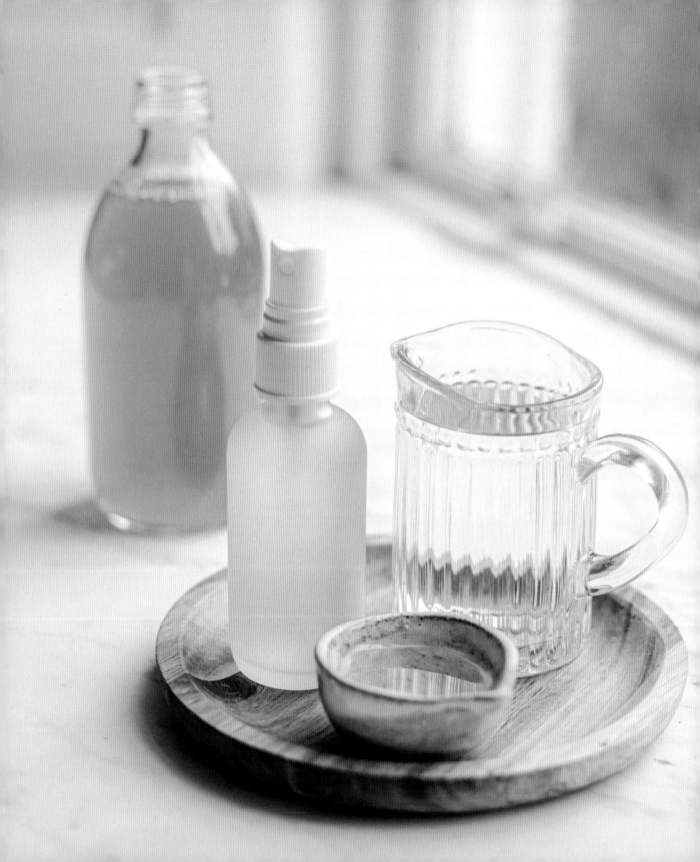

Toners

Botanical toners are for skin what herbal tea is for the body. Toners deliver hydration, nutrients, antioxidants, vitamins, essential oils and health benefits deep into the inner layers of the skin.

For any skin condition that you're facing—whether it's heat and inflammation, dryness, lackluster skin or acne—there is an herb that can provide the support the skin needs.

Making a toner is a way of processing the herbs to make their health benefits available to your skin. My favorite toner to make is the Stovetop Hydrosol (page 40); a traditional skin-care maker in Bali taught me the recipe, and it requires just a soup pot, water, ice and fresh whole food ingredients.

I recommend the Apple Cider Vinegar Toner (page 51) to anyone who needs to stimulate a change in their skin, whether it's clearing acne and breakouts, brightening dull skin or soothing inflammation. The Witch Hazel Toner (page 55) is the perfect medium in which to infuse herbs and botanicals; it's a wonderful astringent that supports toned and clear skin.

Stovetop Hydrosol

A hydrosol is the distillation of botanicals, also called "floral waters." One of the more common hydrosols is rose water, although most of what's sold in the market is not a true hydrosol but actually just water and essential oils. Hydrosols are much more than that! They are made through a process of distillation—simmering plant matter and capturing the condensed steam. A hydrosol includes water-soluble nutrients, vitamins and plant acids, as well as aromatic molecules. Although to the eye a hydrosol looks like plain water, it's actually active and alive with healing constituents.

The scent of hydrosols is not like essential oils—they smell more of the plant matter, like an herbal tea. Yet hydrosols can be used as aromatherapy because they contain aromatic molecules that, when inhaled, travel to the physical centers of the brain that stimulate a mood-altering effect.

This recipe teaches you how to make a hydrosol on your stove. You can use fresh herbs like basil, mint and rosemary. Fragrant flowers make beautiful hydrosols, as well as fragrant greens such as the leaves of a lime tree—I've even used the needles from my Christmas tree! From your kitchen, you can use scraps like the rinds of citrus or even vegetables, each bringing their own benefits, scent and properties. Feel inspired and get creative!

Skin type: all skin types | ***Shelf life:*** 6 months

About 2 cups (50 g) botanicals of choice (fresh, not dried)

About 6 cups (1.5 L) drinking water (tap or bottled)

Roughly 8 cups (1.8 kg) ice cubes

Get a steamer pot with two tiers; the bottom tier is where you will simmer the botanicals in water. It will look like you're making soup! The top tier is where you will place a bowl to collect the hydrosol. As the steam travels up, it will hit the cool lid, condense into liquid and drip into the bowl. It's important that the collection bowl sits separate from the water, so that you're only collecting the distilled water (hydrosol), not the simmering water.

If you don't have a steamer pot, you can use a large soup pot with a metal rack (or upside-down bowl) inside to elevate the collection bowl above the simmering water.

Once you have your setup, you are ready to make the hydrosol. Place the fresh botanicals in the pot. Cover the ingredients with water, and place the pot on the stove over medium heat.

If you're using a two-tiered steamer pot, place the top tier into the pot and put a heatproof bowl in the center. If you're using a rack or upside-down bowl, place those over the water and then put a heatproof bowl on top. For either setup, put the lid on the pot upside down. This will guide the water to drip down into the center, falling into the bowl.

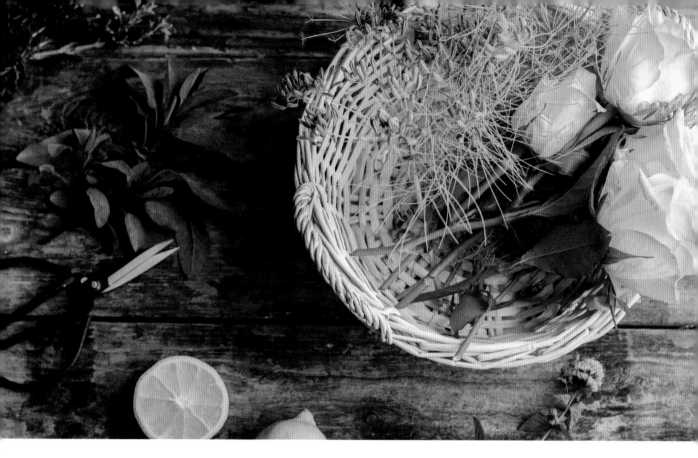

On top of the upside-down lid, place a plastic baggie full of ice cubes. This will keep the lid cool, so that when the steam hits it, it will condense into a liquid. If you don't have an ice maker that will make large amounts of ice cubes, purchase a bag of ice at the supermarket, or the night before you plan to make your hydrosol, freeze water in a large container to make a block of ice.

Allow the water and botanicals to simmer, gently, for 30 minutes. Throughout that time, you'll need to pour out the ice as it melts on top of the pot and add fresh ice. Always keep the lid cool.

You will see the hydrosol collecting in the bowl, giving you about ½ cup (120 ml) in 30 minutes.

Remove the bowl carefully and pour the hydrosol into a sterilized spritz bottle.

You can use your hydrosol right away, but it does take 24 to 48 hours for the hydrosol to settle and the scent to develop.

TIP: Spray hydrosol on your skin, in the air or on your linens. It's safe and gentle enough for babies, people with sensitive skin and the elderly.

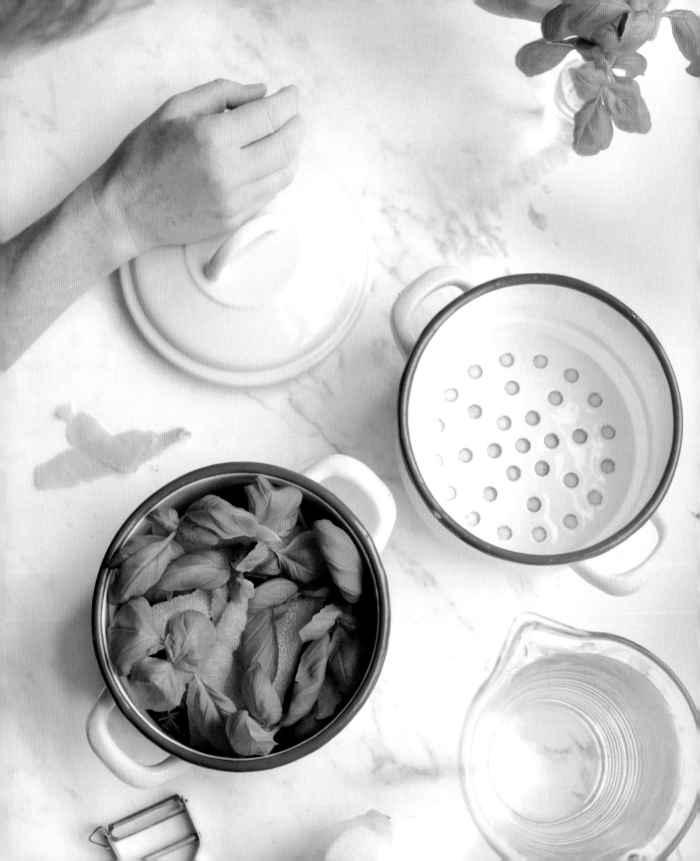

Clean & Clear Hydrosol Toner

This hydrosol features basil, a powerful antibacterial that promotes clear skin, with balancing lemon peel to help control oil production. The combination smells clean and refreshing and helps keep skin clear of bacteria that causes breakouts. Use this hydrosol as a toner, daily after cleansing and before applying your Facial Serum (page 71).

Skin type: oily, acne-prone skin | ***Shelf life:*** 6 months

---

2 cups (48 g) fresh basil leaves

Rind of 2 lemons

About 6 cups (1.5 L) drinking water (tap or bottled)

Roughly 8 cups (1.8 kg) ice cubes

Place the basil leaves and lemon rind in the water, and follow the Stovetop Hydrosol instructions (pages 40–41).

To use, spray your skin liberally and use a cotton pad to swipe clean. This will clean and freshen skin. Then mist again and allow the hydrosol to soak into your skin. Always massage a few drops of oil (such as the Facial Serum, page 71) into your skin after allowing the hydrosol to soak in to lock in the hydration of the hydrosol.

The aromatherapy is clarifying and mood-uplifting but also calming. It's a great way to both start and end the day!

TIPS: I find it more economical to purchase a whole basil plant from the supermarket, rather than buy the little packets of fresh herbs. Basil can grow indoors by a sunny window. If you harvest the plant carefully, you'll get new leaves growing for your next batch!

If you drink lemon water in the morning or use lemons in your kitchen, make use of the leftover peels and turn them into a hydrosol! Save money, and make more from less!

Comfort Hydrosol Toner

This hydrosol toner is a wash of relief for sensitive skin. It features herbs traditionally used to soothe chronic inflammation, like acne or eczema, and even acute inflammation, like sunburn. Aloe calms irritated skin, cucumber cools heat and lemon balm supports healing. The aromatherapy and nervine actions of lemon balm also play a big role in healing, soothing the nervous system and reducing stress.

Skin type: all skin types, especially irritated skin | ***Shelf life:*** 6 months

1 aloe leaf, homegrown or from a supermarket

2 cups (48 g) lemon balm

1 cucumber, sliced

About 6 cups (1.5 L) drinking water (tap or bottled)

Roughly 8 cups (1.8 kg) ice cubes

Place the aloe, lemon balm and cucumber in the water, and follow the Stovetop Hydrosol instructions (pages 40–41).

To use, spray your skin liberally, allowing the hydrosol to soak in well. Mist throughout the day as needed. Always finish with a few drops of oil massaged over your skin to lock in hydration. You can also keep this in the refrigerator to use as a cooling after-sun spray or a cooling facial mist to freshen and wake up your skin.

TIP: Purchase a lemon balm plant from your local gardening supply store or nursery. Carefully trim and harvest the leaves; more will grow for the next batch.

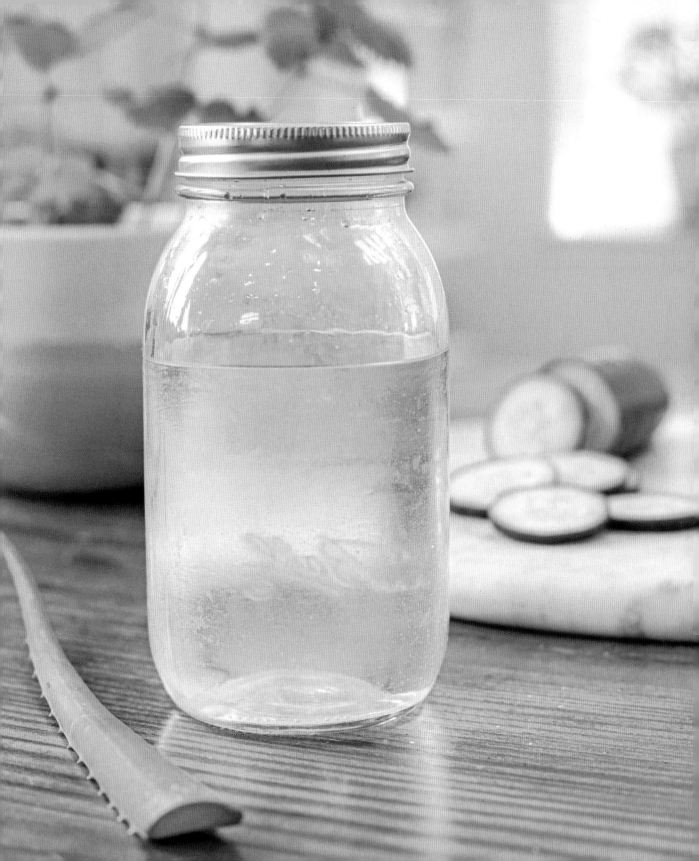

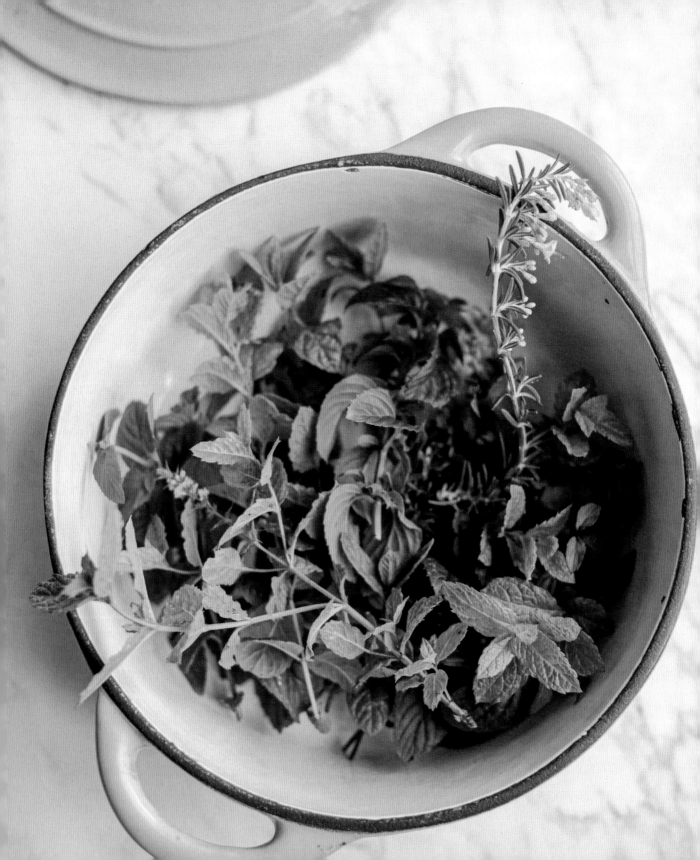

Rejuvenate Hydrosol Toner

This blend wakes up tired skin and promotes circulation to oxygenate skin cells. Inhalation of the hydrosol also helps with respiratory issues, to open up breathing. Both rosemary and peppermint are loaded with antioxidant, antimicrobial and anti-inflammatory properties. This blend beats fatigue and stress in the body and in the mind, leaving you feeling refreshed and restored.

Skin type: all skin types, especially dull or congested skin | ***Shelf life:*** 6 months

---

2 cups (48 g) mint leaves

Handful of rosemary sprigs

About 6 cups (1.5 L) drinking water (tap or bottled)

Roughly 8 cups (1.8 kg) ice cubes

Place the mint leaves and rosemary in the water, and follow the Stovetop Hydrosol instructions (pages 40–41).

To use, spray liberally over your skin, allowing the hydrosol to soak in well. Mist in the mornings, instead of using water to cleanse. Spray your skin with hydrosol and swipe clean with a cotton pad. Mist your skin again before you apply your Facial Serum (page 71); this will give your skin the full moisturization it needs.

TIP: Rosemary and mint have a stimulating effect, traditionally used to promote hair growth. Use this toner on your hair, spraying all over and making sure to work it into your scalp.

Fragrant Hydrosol Toner

This blend smells amazing! It's so fragrant and delicious, you'll want to mist it everywhere! And because hydrosols are gentle and safe, you can use it as often and liberally as you want. This is what I consider a therapeutic fragrance—it combines herbalism and aromatherapy. The citrus in the blend helps to clarify skin; it has potent antibacterial properties and uplifts the mood, finishing with a warm and intoxicating vanilla touch.

Skin type: all skin types | ***Shelf life:*** 6 months

Peel of 1 orange

Peel of 1 grapefruit

Peel of 1 lemon

Peel of 1 lime

½ tsp vanilla extract

About 6 cups (1.5 L) drinking water (tap or bottled)

Roughly 8 cups (1.8 kg) ice cubes

Place the orange, grapefruit, lemon and lime peels and vanilla in the water, and follow the Stovetop Hydrosol instructions (pages 40–41).

To use, spray liberally all over your skin and clothes and in the air. You can also mist your hair—this blend makes a nourishing and softening hair fragrance.

After you mist your skin with a hydrosol, it's always a good idea to follow with two to three drops of oil to lock in the hydration—try the Facial Serum (page 71). You could also use the Creamy Cleansing Balm (page 26), which is a multipurpose product and can double as a moisturizer.

TIP: When you peel the rinds, use the fruit to make an herbal lemonade, combining the fruit with water and lavender-infused honey (see Herbal-Infused Honey 101 on page 22) to taste.

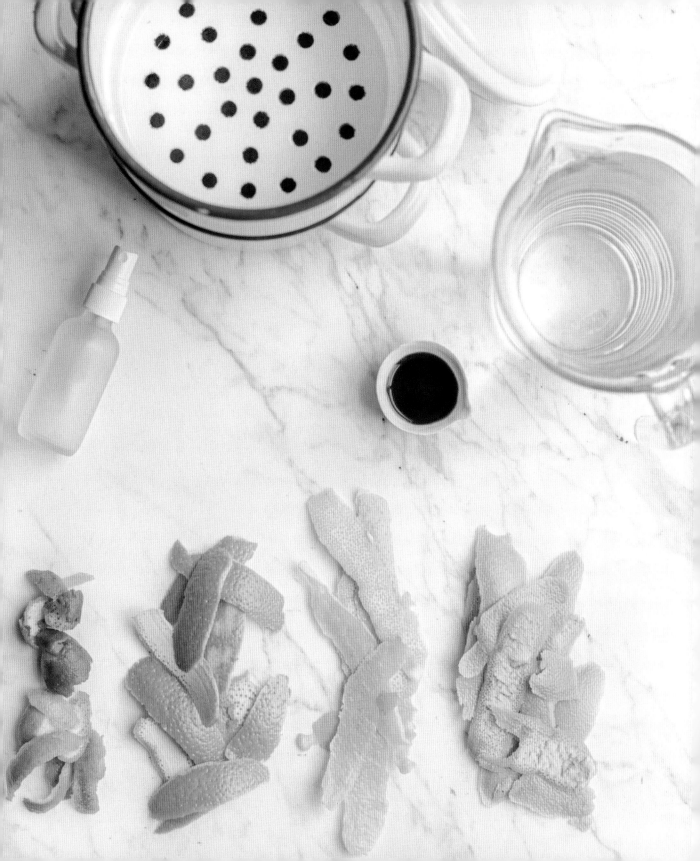

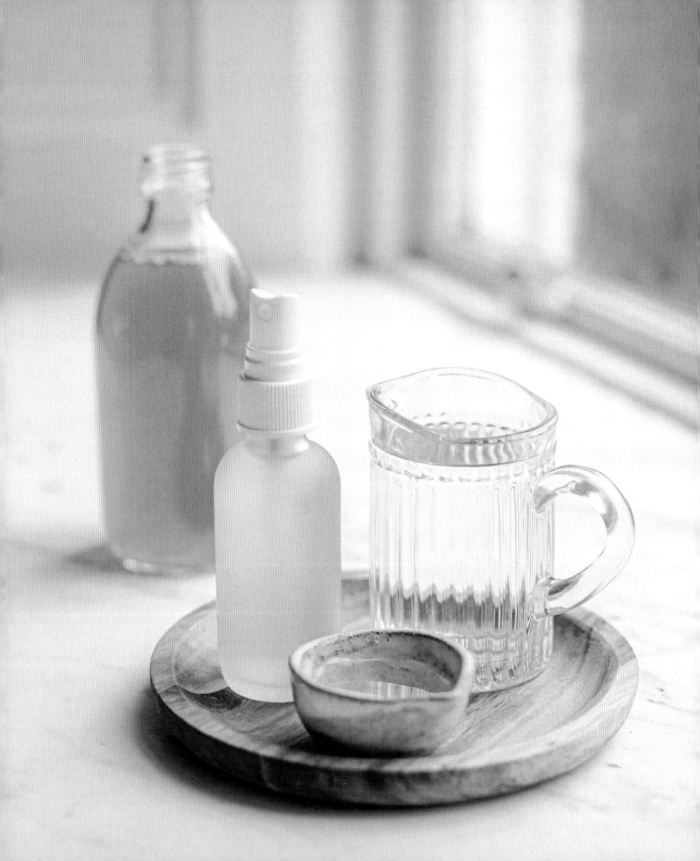

Apple Cider Vinegar Toner

If you can get past the scent of vinegar, I promise you will be in love with the effects of this toner. Being so inexpensive and easily accessible, apple cider vinegar is one of the most effective skin-care ingredients I have found. It balances skin, promotes cell turnover, decongests pores, clears away breakouts and brings down inflammation. Too many recipes I see online use vinegar in high concentrations. Vinegar should always be diluted—it is potent! Through teaching hundreds of people this recipe in my in-person workshops, I have found the perfect dilution that is both effective but also gentle enough for all skin types.

Skin type: all skin types | ***Shelf life:*** 2 weeks

2 tsp (10 ml) jojoba oil

10 drops lavender essential oil

2 tbsp (30 ml) raw apple cider vinegar (see Tips)

½ cup (120 ml) water

Clean a 4-ounce (120-ml) glass spray bottle with boiling water, and spray rubbing alcohol through it to clean the spray pump. When the bottle is clean and dry, add the jojoba oil and lavender essential oil. Swirl together, then add the apple cider vinegar and top off with the water.

To use, first remove makeup with the Makeup Melt Cleansing Oil (page 17). Before each use, shake the bottle to disperse the oils and vinegar and then spray your skin liberally. Let it sit for a minute or two. Soak a cotton pad in water and squeeze out the excess water, then swipe your face clean with the cotton pad.

This blend already includes moisturizing oils to keep your skin soft and nourished, but if needed, you can finish with a few drops of Facial Serum (page 71).

TIPS: When purchasing your apple cider vinegar, choose a brand that includes the "mother" for the active benefits.

Don't worry about the scent—it goes away quickly!

Infused Vinegar

Vinegar has long been used as a menstruum to extract beneficial properties from plants. It extracts tannins, which have a toning effect on skin. It draws out water-soluble vitamins, and the acidic nature of vinegar is especially good at drawing out minerals, which helps to strengthen connective tissues. The stimulating actions of plants are enhanced by vinegar, making them beneficial as skin care. Infused vinegars are used internally and externally, to augment beauty and health. They're incredibly easy and inexpensive to make, and for the benefits they bring, it's worth it!

In this recipe, we're making a mineral-rich, vitamin C–rich blend with nettles and rose.

Skin type: all skin types | **Shelf life:** 6 months

¼ cup (6 g) dried nettles

¼ cup (9 g) dried rose petals

1–2 cups (240–480 ml) apple cider vinegar

Add the nettles and rose petals to your jar, and pour in the vinegar until the herbs have been fully covered, with 1 to 2 inches (3 to 5 cm) of space on top. If the lid of the jar is metal, place a piece of parchment paper over the mouth of the jar before sealing shut.

Allow the infusion to sit for 2 to 4 weeks, shaking the jar every few days to help the infusion process, and then strain out the herbs. Store the infused vinegar in a dark cupboard and use it as needed for your recipes. It's especially good to use an infused vinegar in the Apple Cider Vinegar Toner (page 51) and the Clarifying Hair Rinse (page 141).

I also love pouring 1 cup (240 ml) of this infused vinegar into a bath to soothe sunburns and stressed skin. While it may sound counterintuitive to use acidic vinegar to soothe, it actually has an anti-inflammatory and healing effect on the skin and helps to restore and rebalance the skin's acid mantle.

TIP: Vinegar extracts essential oils, so add aromatic herbs to your blend to enhance the aroma. Try peppermint, rosemary or dried lemon peels.

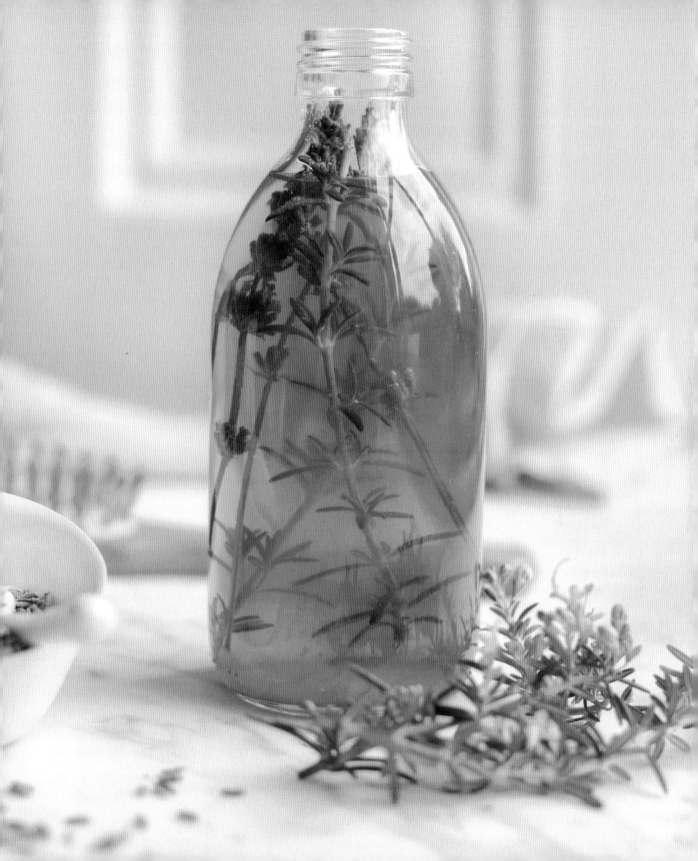

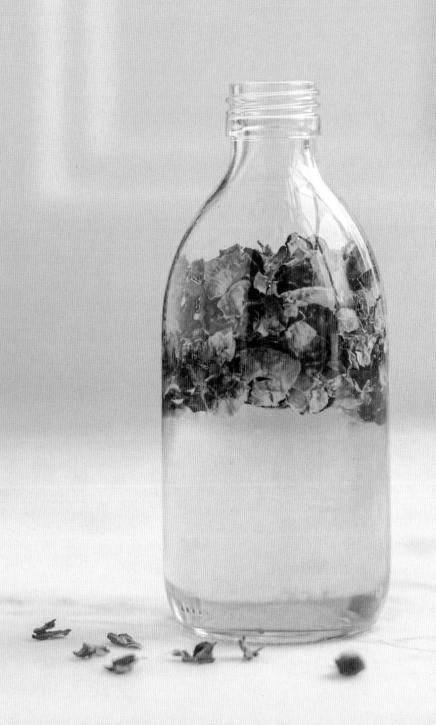

Witch Hazel Toner

I recommend this toner for oily skin—it's amazing at helping to clear up breakouts and rebalance oil production. Dry and normal skin types may find it to be drying over time, because witch hazel has 14 percent alcohol. But it's the alcohol content that makes witch hazel a good menstruum to extract the beneficial properties of herbs. Use this toner to clear acne as needed. For some people, it can be used daily; for others, it may only be a protocol until the skin clears. The astringent action of witch hazel is also good at toning the skin and reducing inflammation.

Skin type: acne-prone or oily skin | **Shelf life:** 6 months

---

Dried rose petals or herb of choice (calendula is a great choice for acne-prone skin)

Witch hazel made only of witch hazel extract and up to 14% alcohol

Choose a glass jar with a lid, sized to match the amount of product you want to make; you will want to fill the jar fully with the herbs and witch hazel, not leaving an air gap. I always prefer to start with a small batch.

Add the herbs to the jar, filling the jar halfway. Pour in the witch hazel to fully cover the herbs, filling the jar all the way to the top. And that's it! Let the jar sit for 2 to 4 weeks, and give it a shake every couple of days to encourage the extraction.

Always label your infusion with a date so you know when it's time to strain out the herbs. Leave yourself a calendar reminder, so that you won't forget!

When it's ready, strain out the herbs and reserve the infused witch hazel in a glass bottle. Keep it by your sink so you can use it as needed.

To use, apply it directly onto the skin with a cotton pad; you don't need to dilute it. You can apply it all over your face or just over areas where you see pimples or that need extra cleansing. Do not wipe off the witch hazel—allow it to soak into your skin and do its work!

TIP: Use this toner as a hand sanitizer by adding antimicrobial herbs and essential oils like lavender or tea tree.

Steamer Tabs

Steaming helps the skin to release any congestion it might be holding, and it opens the pores to better absorb all of the nutrients from the serums, masks and products that follow. Steaming stimulates circulation and gives the skin a healthy, rosy glow. When you make these Steamer Tabs, you can just pop one in a bowl of hot water and steam away!

Skin type: all skin types | **Shelf life:** 6 months

---

1 cup (220 g) baking soda

½ cup (115 g) citric acid

10 drops sage essential oil

10 drops lavender essential oil

1 tbsp (3 g) dried lavender buds

Rubbing alcohol in a spray bottle

Find a mold to press the Steamer Tabs into; I use a silicone muffin pan.

In a large bowl, mix the baking soda and citric acid together. Add in the essential oils and mix well to fully combine. Add the lavender buds and stir to mix.

Lightly mist the mixture with rubbing alcohol, making sure not to use too much; you don't want the mixture too wet. Continue to mist and work the mixture with your hands just until it can clump up and hold its shape.

Press the mixture into the molds, aiming for approximately ¼ cup (60 g) for each Steamer Tab, and let it sit for a few minutes. Pop them out and let them air dry on the counter for 24 hours. Setting them on a cooling rack is ideal, so that they get air on all sides to dry them fully.

To use, start with clean skin. Remove all makeup with the Makeup Melt Cleansing Oil (page 17). Fill a large bowl with boiling water. Add a Steamer Tab to the water and quickly place a towel over your head. Sit with your face over the bowl, at a far enough distance that the steam doesn't burn, and let the fragrant steam wash over your skin. As the steam and essential oils deeply cleanse your skin, the aromatherapy also plays an important role in helping to calm the nervous system and reduce feelings of anxiety. Breathe in deeply.

Steam for 5 to 7 minutes and then immediately proceed with the next steps of your routine, either applying a serum or a mask treatment.

TIP: You can also use Steamer Tabs in your bath and enjoy the hot water as a "steaming" treatment. Steamer Tabs also work in the shower—just place one on the floor of the shower to enjoy the aromatherapy!

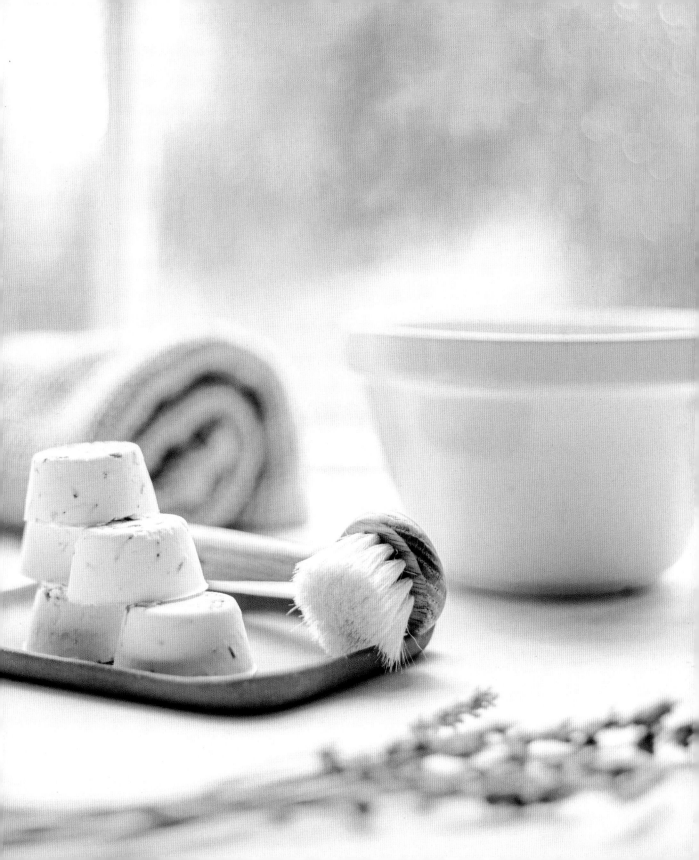

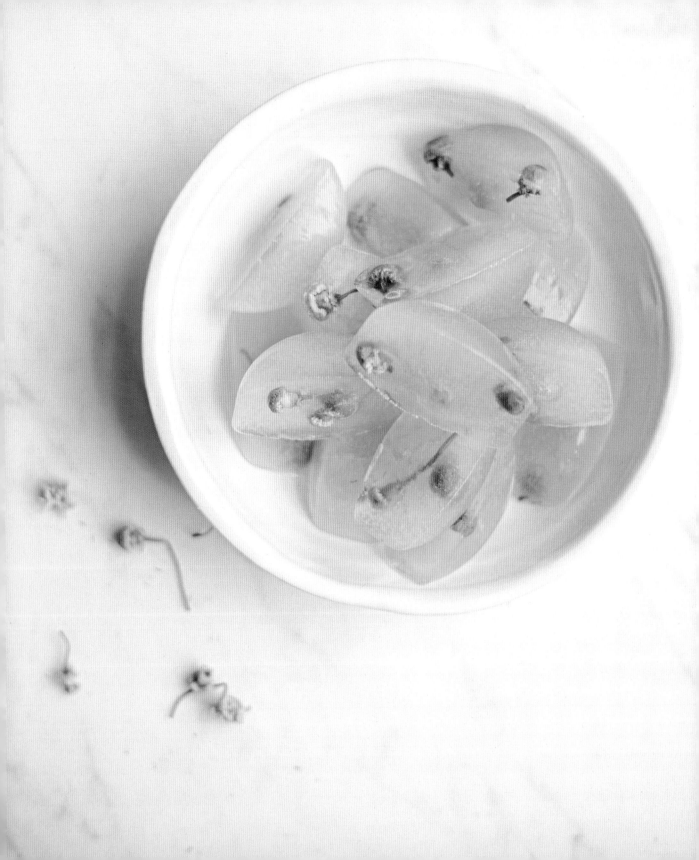

Chamomile Ice

Audrey Hepburn famously said her secret to youthful vibrant skin was washing her face every day with cold water. As we age, our natural functions like cell turnover can begin to slow down. A cold touch has a very stimulating effect on the skin, and just like a cold shower, it wakes you up and jump-starts a healthy glow! It helps to take the redness out of pimples and reduces swelling and puffiness around the eyes and face. If you can stand the cold, the benefits will be well worth it!

Skin type: all skin types | *Shelf life:* 3 months

1½ cups (360 ml) bottled water

4 tbsp (12 g) dried chamomile, plus more for sprinkling

Start by making yourself a very strong chamomile tea. Boil the water in a kettle. Add the chamomile to a mug or small bowl, and cover with the hot water from the kettle. Let the tea sit for 10 minutes and then strain. (This would be too strong and bitter to drink but is perfect for our skin-care needs.) Let the tea cool slightly as you prepare your ice-cube tray. Add a sprinkling of chamomile to each chamber of the tray, then pour in the herbal tea.

Set the tray in the freezer. When the cubes are completely frozen, pop them out and store in an airtight freezer container. Make sure the container is labeled!

To use, fill a bowl with 1 cup (240 ml) of cool water and add two ice cubes, letting them melt. Soak a soft cloth in this ice-cold herbal water. Squeeze out excess water and place the cloth over your skin as a compress for 10 seconds. Repeat several times.

You can also dunk your face directly in the bowl of herbal ice water, as many times as you can, to de-puff your skin and instantly look more awake! This is so good in the mornings or when you want glowing skin.

Alternatively, you can run an herbal ice cube over your face. If you do this, use only the frozen chamomile tea; do not add the extra dry herbs before freezing or they could scratch your skin. Perform "ice sculpting," running the ice cube along your cheekbones and jawline.

TIP: Add these ice cubes to a glass of water to make yourself a delicious iced tea!

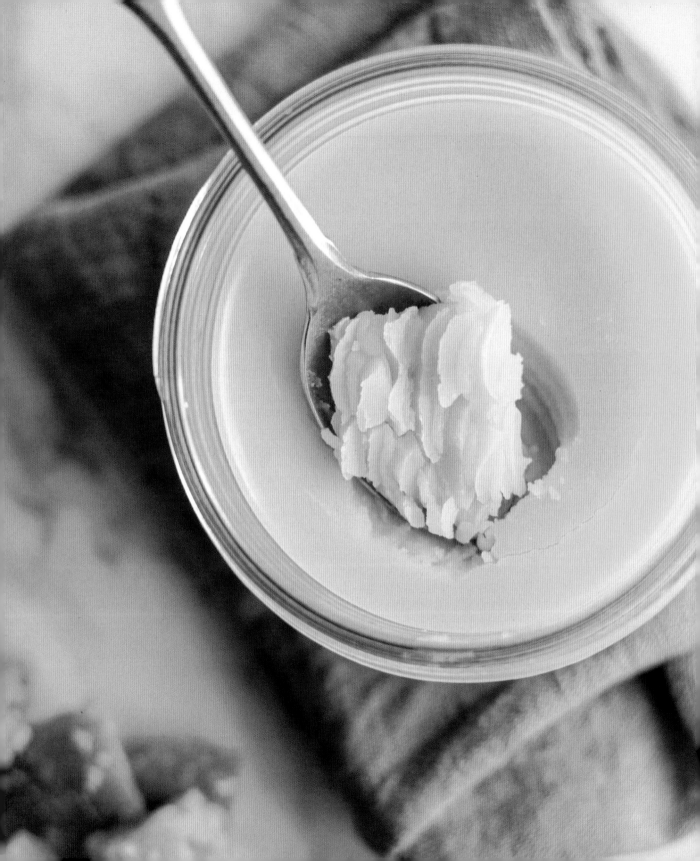

Moisturizers

The skin produces sebum, our own natural oil that keeps the skin lubricated and flexible. If you imagine skin cells as bricks, sebum is the mortar that fills in the gaps. It holds hydration in and keeps bacteria and irritants out. Plants also produce oils that, in many ways, are chemically similar to our own—they're made of fatty acids and phytonutrients, which the skin recognizes as nourishment. When you apply plant oil to the skin, it becomes part of your skin structure, strengthening and supporting every cell.

The biggest question around oils is knowing how to choose the right oil for your skin type. With hundreds of options, it can be overwhelming! I've found the most success with jojoba oil; it is structurally very similar to our own sebum and works well for different skin types. When I teach workshops, I always work with jojoba oil, because I know it will suit everyone in the group.

Jojoba is perfectly suited to be your total head-to-toe moisturizer and is a star ingredient in some of my favorite products in this chapter. You can find it in the Citrus Blender Lotion (page 63), Healing Balm (page 68), Sunrise Body Oil (page 76) and many other moisturizers.

The richer moisturizers, like the Tasty Lip Balm (page 67) and Healing Balm (page 68) are made with oils and butters. Butters protect the skin barrier and are especially good for very dry skin and for protecting skin inflamed from conditions like eczema and psoriasis.

For all of the recipes, I focus on just three different types of butters: shea, mango and cocoa.

Shea butter stimulates circulation and oxygenates the skin. Mango butter is an astringent. It controls oil protection and has a very unique feature: when it soaks in, the skin is dry to the touch. Cocoa butter is an occlusive—it does not readily soak in. It actually coats the skin and protects against water loss, which makes it ideal for skin that needs extra protection. Both shea butter and mango butter are lightweight and can be used head-to-toe, but cocoa butter is very rich, and I recommend using it only for the body.

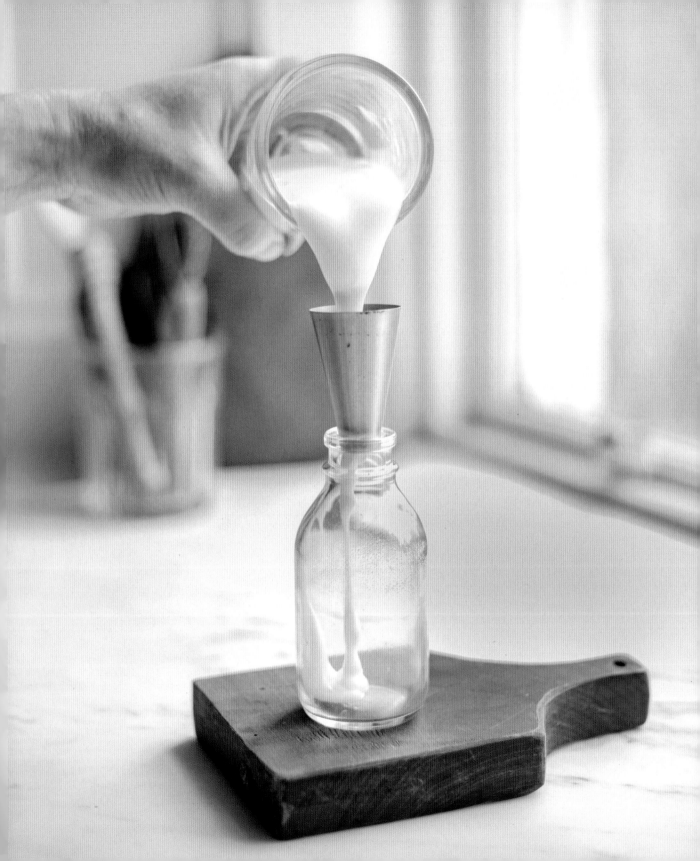

Citrus Blender Lotion

Oils and butters are always good for the skin, but sometimes you want a moisturizer that feels hydrating and lightweight. What you want is lotion! This recipe combines hydrosol with moisturizing oils, binding them together through a process called emulsification. Think about using an herbal-infused oil (pages 18–19) and different hydrosols (pages 40–48) to create a specialized lotion.

Skin type: all skin types | ***Shelf life:*** 2 weeks, or 1 month in the refrigerator

---

3 tsp (9 g) grated beeswax

¼ cup (60 ml) jojoba oil

24 drops sweet orange essential oil

¼ cup (60 ml) fragrant hydrosol, or aloe vera jelly (see Tip)

TIP: Use hydrosol as the liquid base, which has an acidic pH and greater shelf life than plain water. Or you can use a natural aloe vera jelly, which is preserved with citric acid (found in health-food stores).

Over medium heat, bring a small saucepan of water to a simmer. Set a heatproof bowl over the pot, add the beeswax and let it melt. Add the jojoba oil, and if the beeswax congeals a bit when you add the oil, let it sit over the heat until it has fully melted with the oil.

Pour the melted beeswax and oil into a tall measuring cup that is big enough to hold an immersion blender. Add the essential oil as the beeswax begins to cool. The key to lotion is that the oil and hydrosol need to be the same temperature. Let the oil sit until it cools down fully.

When the oil mixture congeals and has a very soft, balm-like texture, you're ready to incorporate the hydrosol. Stick an immersion blender into the jar and begin mixing. With the blender constantly running, very slowly drizzle in the measured hydrosol. Always pour the hydrosol into the oil, not the other way around. The slower the drizzle, the better the chances you'll get it to emulsify and bind with the oil and beeswax.

Continue blending and drizzling in the hydrosol until it's all incorporated and the mixture is creamy. Bottle and use as you would any lotion. When using the lotion, it's important not to contaminate it. Do not scoop into the lotion with your fingers—it's best to use a pump bottle. This recipe is formulated to be a body lotion, but if you also want to use it on your face, cut the essential oils to just 12 drops.

You can keep this lotion at room temperature in your bathroom or on a bedside table for easy use, but make sure to use it up within 2 weeks. If you store it in the refrigerator, the lotion will be nice and cool, which helps to stimulate and tighten the skin. You can use up extra lotion by doing a deep conditioning hair mask treatment—or slather your feet with it and put on socks overnight for the softest feet ever!

Solid Body Moisturizer

Made with emollient-rich butters, solid lotions are immensely moisturizing and leave your skin feeling touchably soft. Used all over your body, or anywhere that needs a little extra care, the butters melt over the warmth of the skin and penetrate as you massage them in. A solid lotion is very easy to use and travel with and is incredibly fun to make.

Skin type: all skin types	***Shelf life:*** 6 months

¼ cup (56 g) cocoa butter

¼ cup (56 g) shea butter

TIP: Cocoa butter has a strong chocolaty aroma. Enjoy it just as it is, or use the "refined" version for a neutral scent, then add 20 to 40 drops of an essential oil of your choice.

Over medium heat, bring a small saucepan of water to a simmer. Set a heatproof bowl over the pot and add about half of the cocoa butter to the bowl. Stir it continuously as it begins to melt. When it is melted, add the remaining cocoa butter and the shea butter.

Continue melting the mixture over a very gentle simmer, stirring continuously for another 5 minutes. Then take it off the heat and let it cool slightly before pouring into a mold. I prefer to use silicone muffin molds—the finished product will pop out easily, and the size is perfect for a handheld solid moisturizer. I've also used mini loaf pans and even ice-cube trays. This recipe makes one large bar or two smaller bars. Do note that the larger the size, the longer it takes to harden. Put the mold in the freezer for about 15 minutes, or until it feels hard to the touch. Larger bars may need up to 30 minutes to solidify.

Take the mold out and pop out the solid lotion. Let it sit at room temperature to allow the cocoa butter to fully harden. Do not rush this; give the bar at least 12 hours to fully harden. It may feel too soft or melt if you try using it straightaway, so don't touch it until it's firm and ready.

This recipe has no beeswax to keep the bar hard, because beeswax takes away the creaminess. Adding more cocoa butter will keep the bar hard, but it can make this bar feel a little greasy. This recipe may produce a softer bar, especially if you live in a hot climate like I do. After giving it 12 hours to set, if you feel it is still too soft, take the soft bar and begin to roll it in your hands, gently compressing the bar and changing the shape. Set it down for another hour to harden again—and then, like magic, it sets into the perfect texture, firm yet creamy.

To use, glide the bar over your skin. The butters melt over the warmth of your body and soak right in. It's especially good during pregnancy to prevent stretch marks and for rubbing over patches of eczema to soothe and protect. You can apply this balm to your face, but do so sparingly, as the cocoa butter can be quite rich. It's wonderful for the lips!

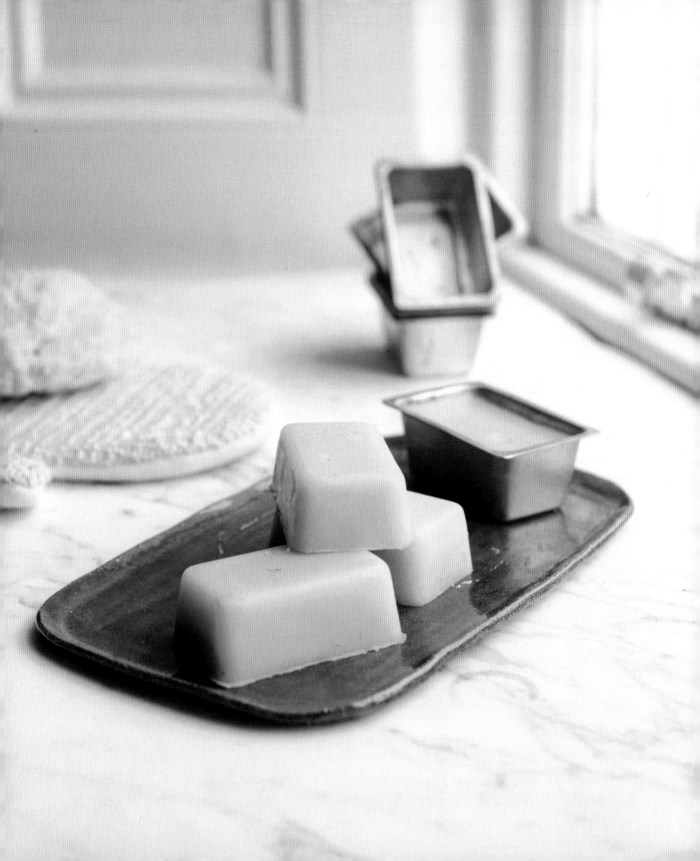

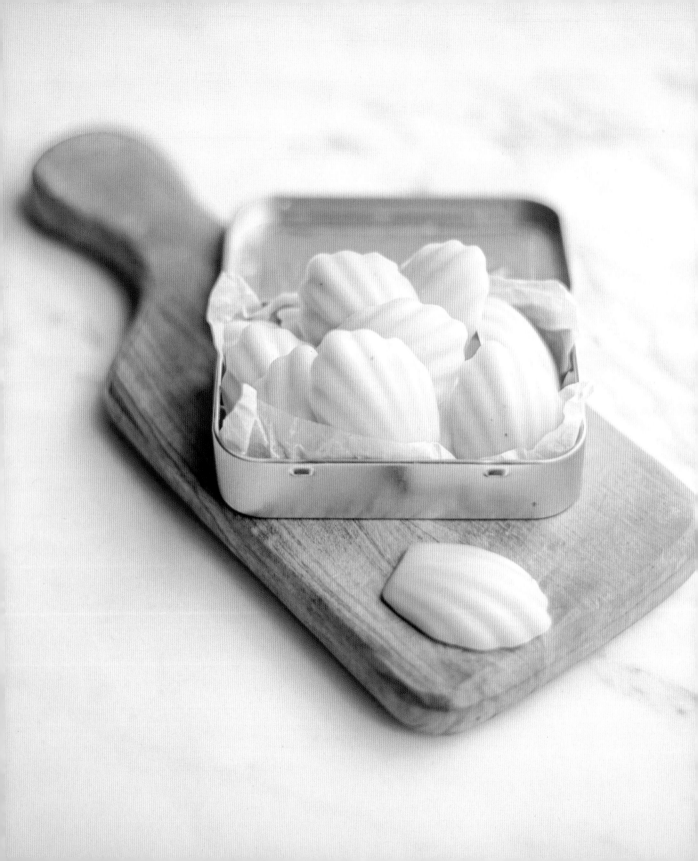

Tasty Lip Balm

Make your lips feel deliciously soft with flavored lip balms. This balm is made with conditioning shea and mango butters and a touch of beeswax to protect your lips from becoming chapped. The recipe includes candy flavoring, which comes in nearly every flavor you can imagine! My girls love soda-pop flavors, like cola. I'm a huge fan of caramel and green apple, my favorite candy flavors!

Skin type: all skin types | ***Shelf life:*** 6 months

---

1 tbsp (14 g) beeswax

1 tbsp (14 g) shea butter

1 tbsp (14 g) mango butter

⅛–¼ tsp candy flavoring (see Tip)

Over medium heat, bring a small saucepan of water to a simmer. Set a heatproof bowl over the pot, and add the beeswax and let it melt. When the beeswax has melted, add the shea and mango butters. When the butters are melted, add the candy flavoring. Stir well to combine. Smell and taste a drop of the melted mixture over your lips (cooling it slightly first—it will be hot), and if you need to, add a little more flavoring.

Remove the mixture from the heat and pour into a mold. You can make a package-free lip balm by pouring the mixture into a small mold, like a silicone ice-cube tray or chocolate mold. Or purchase lip balm tubes online (look for cardboard tubes for an eco-friendly option). Allow the lip balms to sit out on a counter for a few hours. Sometimes butters can crystallize when melted and then reharden too quickly in the refrigerator. If you can't wait, let it harden naturally at room temperature for an hour, then complete the hardening process in the refrigerator.

TIP: Make sure to purchase a candy flavoring that is alcohol free, made with glycerine. Look in the baking or spice sections of your supermarket or online.

Healing Balm

When you need deep healing for cracked skin, heels, elbows or lips—or if you have eczema, an itchy rash, extreme dryness or irritation causing you bother—this is the recipe for you. The recipe begins with a base of calendula oil, which is the key to the healing action. Shea butter envelops your skin, and beeswax holds everything together. You'll notice this balm is rich and thick—it forms a barrier of protection wherever you apply it. Yet it's nongreasy—you won't even feel it's there, but it will be silently working to heal and soothe, repair and restore.

Skin type: all skin types, especially skin in need of healing | ***Shelf life:*** 6 months

---

2 tbsp (28 g) beeswax

2 tbsp (28 g) shea butter

¼ cup (60 ml) calendula-infused jojoba oil (see Herbal-Infused Oil 101, pages 18–19)

As with all recipes that call for beeswax, begin by melting the beeswax. It takes the longest to melt, and we want to minimize the amount of heat that our butters and oils are exposed to.

Over medium heat, bring a small saucepan of water to a simmer. Set a heatproof bowl over the pot, and add the beeswax and let it melt. When the beeswax has fully melted, add the shea butter. The shea butter will melt over the residual heat, so you can turn off the stove. When the shea butter is melted, add the calendula-infused jojoba oil.

Pour the mixture into a 4-oz (120-ml) widemouthed container that you can easily dip into. Let it sit on the counter for a few hours to harden. This balm is really good to travel with and can be used on scratches, rashes or sunburn, so you might want to make a small travel size. I like to use small tin containers used for lip balm that I can easily throw in my bag.

To use, scoop out some balm with your finger and massage it over any area that needs a little extra care and protection, including your face or anywhere head-to-toe. I recommend women use this to massage the breasts, as calendula stimulates the lymphatic system, which clears toxins. You can also use this balm as a nighttime moisturizer. Studies have shown calendula to significantly improve hydration, elasticity and firmness of skin.

TIP: Don't wait until you need it to make this balm. With a shelf life of 6 months, it's a good idea to have a pot of this balm in your home, ready to bring you comfort and healing anytime!

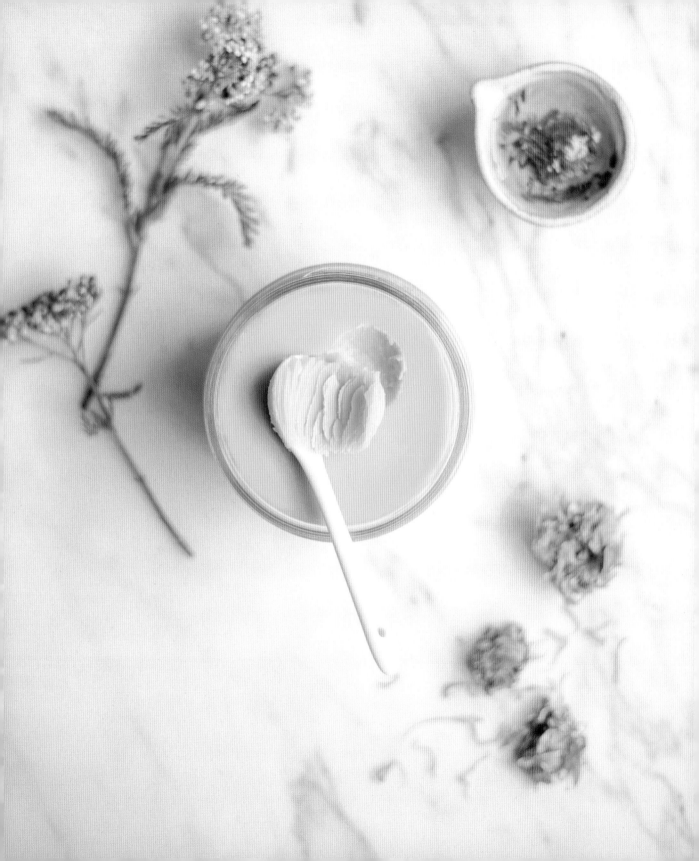

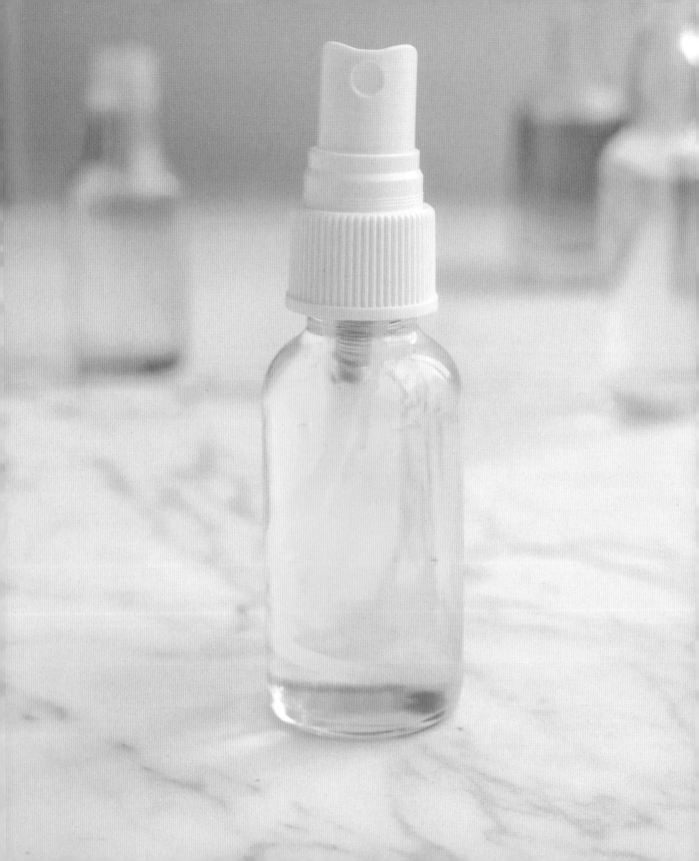

Facial Serum

Serums are a multivitamin for the skin. More than just a moisturizer, a serum provides nutrients to the deep inner layers of your skin for a healthy complexion. Serums should be used daily on damp skin, after your cleanser and toner, but before your moisturizer.

This recipe is my favorite serum blend, with natural sources of papain from papaya seed oil, which decongests pores and promotes cell turnover, and squalene from rice bran oil, which supports plump and hydrated skin. Rosehip brings a big dose of collagen-boosting, skin-brightening vitamin C! This blend soaks in quickly and penetrates deep where it can deliver anti-inflammatory and soothing support to the inner layers of the skin.

Skin type: all skin types | ***Shelf life:*** 6 months

1 tbsp (15 ml) papaya seed oil

1 tbsp (15 ml) rosehip seed oil

1 tbsp (15 ml) rice bran oil

8 drops lavender essential oil

Clean and dry a bottle for storing your serum. Most serums are packaged in bottles with a dropper top, but I prefer to use a spray bottle for my oils.

Pour the papaya seed oil, rosehip seed oil, rice bran oil and lavender essential oil into the bottle, and swirl to combine.

To use, pat two to three drops of oil all over your face, or two to three spritzes if you are using a spray bottle. You might add a little extra to the under-eye area or any laugh lines as part of your evening routine.

TIP: Here is a list of oils that you can use to create your own unique blend:

Oils for acne-prone skin
Grapeseed, passionfruit seed, watermelon

Oils for scarring
Rosehip seed, cucumber, camellia, buriti

Oils for dry skin
Açaí, buriti, papaya seed, macadamia nut

Oils high in vitamin C (antioxidant, collagen and skin brightening)
Blackberry, marula, passionfruit seed, sea buckthorn

Oils for healthy skin aging
Argan, avocado, blackberry, camellia, cranberry

Moisture-Rich Solid Serum

A solid serum works exactly as your oil serum does but in a solid form, which you may find is easier to both travel with and apply on the go. Serums are nutrient dense and, when used daily, can revitalize and transform the health of your skin. I've added a touch of ultra-lightweight, vitamin C-rich mango butter, which never leaves skin feeling oily! This serum will give you such a healthy glow, without any shine. Although this solid serum is formulated for the face, I also recommend you use it on your neck, chest and hands to give care to areas that often get neglected.

Skin type: all skin types, especially dry skin | **Shelf life:** 3-6 months

---

1 tbsp (14 g) beeswax
2 oz (60 ml) Facial Serum (page 71)
1 tbsp (14 g) mango butter

Making a solid serum involves melting beeswax into the oil, but because of the nature of the specialty oils, you do not want to apply too much heat. With a little patience and gentle heat, you will achieve great results!

Over medium heat, bring a small saucepan of water to a simmer. Set a heatproof bowl over the pot, and add the beeswax and let it melt. When it has melted, turn off the heat and pour in the Facial Serum and mango butter. Allow the residual heat to melt everything into a pool of liquid.

Pour the mixture into the mold of choice. I like using large silicone ice-cube trays, which are the perfect size for a facial balm, and the silicone allows the mixture to pop out easily.

Store your balm in a tin container or a jar, or set it on a pretty dish on your bathroom counter.

To use, glide the balm over clean skin. Use your fingers to gently press the oil into your skin.

TIP: Use your Facial Serum guide (page 71) to choose oils that suit your skin's needs. Or if you already have a serum blend you like, you can use that to make this recipe.

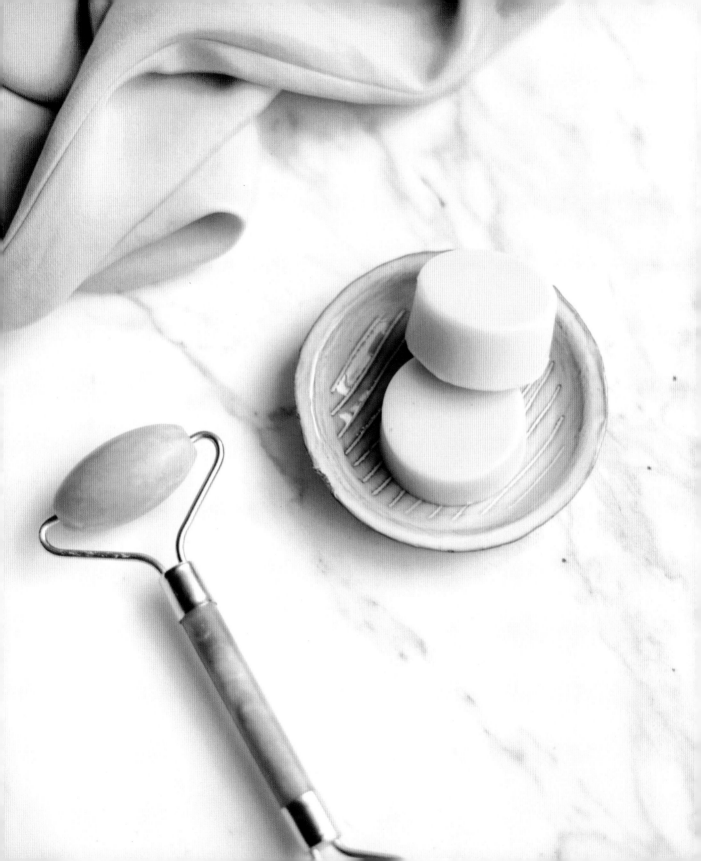

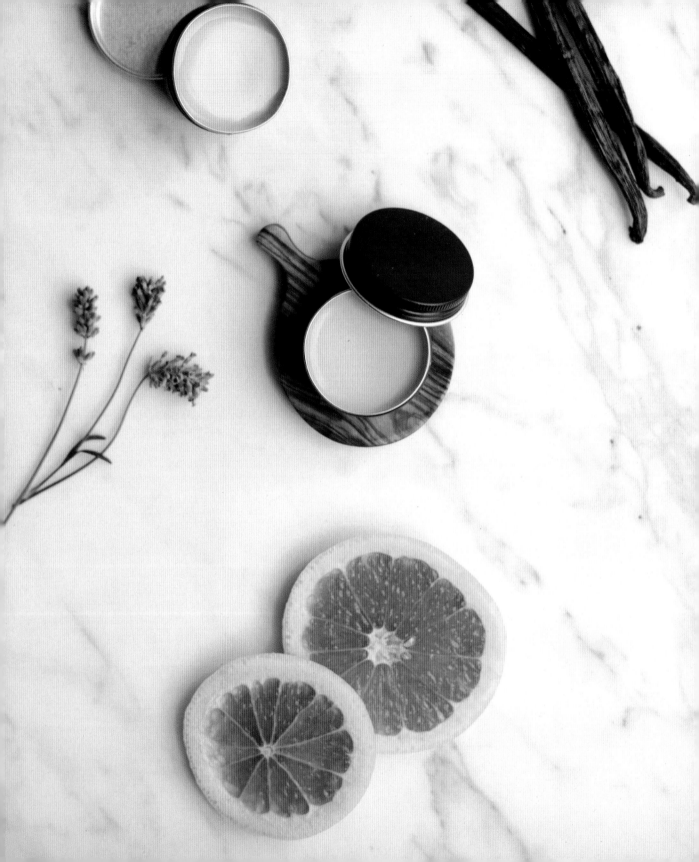

Perfume Balm

I wanted to include this recipe because fragrance is considered to be one of the top allergens. If you are experiencing skin sensitivity or inflammation like acne or eczema, it's important to remove any possible irritants from your routine, like perfume.

This balm uses a higher dilution of essential oils to achieve a beautiful fragrance that also delivers therapeutic benefits! Below I have shared my top three favorite blends.

Spa Luxury—clean and refreshing scent:
8 drops sage + 8 drops lavender essential oils

Citrus Grove—bright and lively scent:
5 drops magnolia + 5 drops white fir + 5 drops grapefruit essential oils

Date Night Dessert—sweet and sexy scent:
8 drops vetiver + 8 drops lime essential oils

Skin types: all skin types | **Shelf life:** 6 months

½ tbsp (7 g) beeswax (refined has no honey scent)

2 tbsp (30 ml) jojoba oil

15–20 drops essential oil

Over medium heat, bring a small saucepan of water to a simmer. Set a heatproof bowl over the pot and add the beeswax and jojoba oil.

Meanwhile, add the essential oils directly into the container that you are using. I recommend a small 1-ounce (30-ml) tin container. When the beeswax and oil are fully melted, pour the mixture into the container with the essential oils.

Allow the balm to cool for a few hours on your kitchen counter, or place in the refrigerator to harden more quickly.

To use, rub your finger into the balm and apply a touch to your pulse points and on the tips of your hair. You can carry this balm with you and reapply as needed.

Sunrise Body Oil

This recipe is a great example of how skin care can be used to support your total well-being, outside and in! Massaging your skin in the morning is a wonderful way to wake up your circulation, activate your lymphatic system and bring energy into your body. It's also going to leave your skin well moisturized and protected all day long. For this body oil, we're using lightweight jojoba, which sinks right in and feels nongreasy. Infused with stimulating calendula, the herbal properties stimulate healing actions in the body. Anti-inflammatory and antioxidant-rich lemongrass also gives a hit of aromatherapy to wake up your mind and your senses and get you set for a good day ahead.

Skin type: all skin types | ***Shelf life:*** 6 months

½ cup (120 ml) calendula-infused jojoba oil (see Herbal-Infused Oil 101, pages 18–19)

30 drops lemongrass essential oil (or any essential oil you find enjoyable and uplifting)

Clean and dry a 4-ounce (120-ml) bottle. You can order a new one online or repurpose one you already have. I like using a spray bottle; I find it so easy to spritz out the oil into the palm of my hand, rather than carefully pouring. But any type of bottle will work.

Pour the calendula-infused jojoba oil into the bottle, then add the lemongrass essential oil.

Swirl the bottle to blend the oils and allow 24 to 48 hours for the scent to settle and develop. For stimulation, rosemary-infused oil is also an excellent choice and blends well with lemongrass essential oil.

To use, massage about 1 teaspoon or about 5 spritzes of oil all over your body. Breathe in the aroma and have yourself a good morning!

TIP: Lemongrass is antibacterial and antifungal. Pour this oil into a footbath to soften and freshen up those feet!

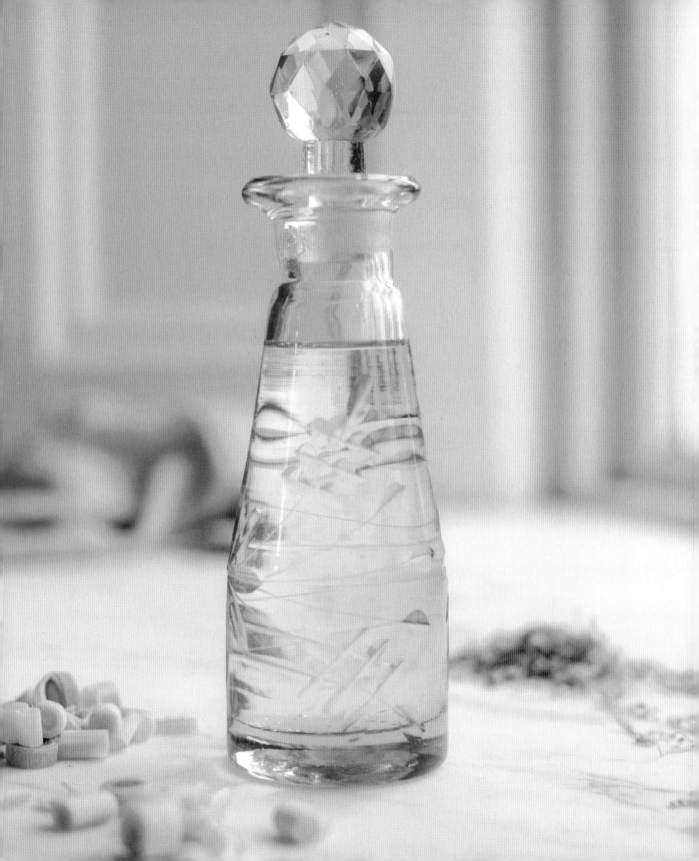

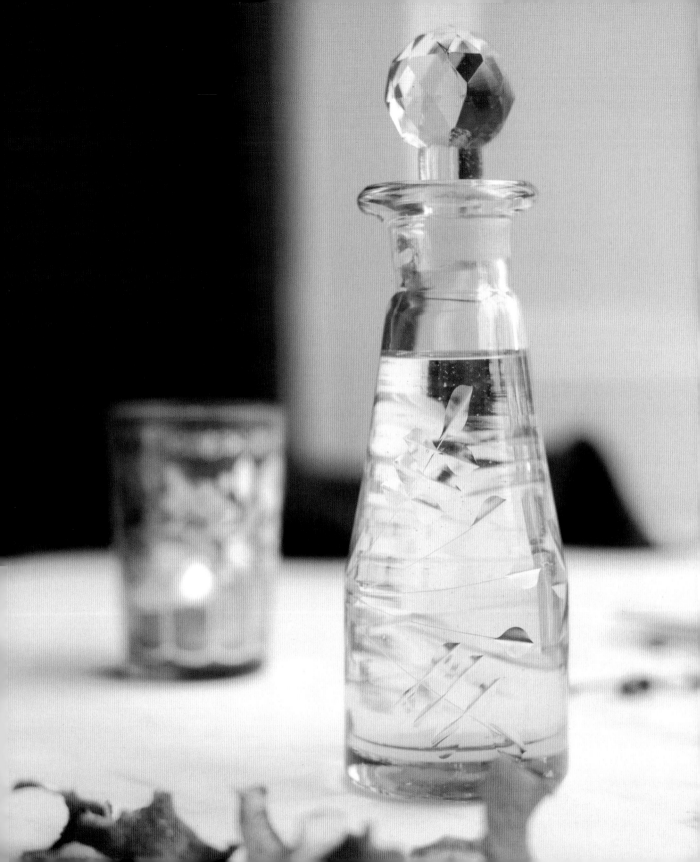

Sunset Body Oil

When it's time to rest and restore, this body oil will take you there. Lavender oil has long been known and enjoyed for its calming effects on the body and mind. It also has been shown to have a positive impact on quality of sleep. Studies show that inhaling lavender as you sleep increases the length of deep sleep, the phase where the heartbeat slows down, muscles relax and the body does its work to heal, detoxify and restore. A touch of sweet orange puts you in a good mood for bedtime, and we're using anti-inflammatory rose in the blend, also known to be an aromatic nervine—rose helps to soothe feelings of stress and anxiety.

Massage your skin with this body oil before bed, and get the quality sleep you need!

Skin type: all skin types | ***Shelf life:*** 6 months

½ cup (120 ml) rose-infused jojoba oil (see Herbal-Infused Oil 101, pages 18–19)

15 drops lavender essential oil (or any essential oil you find enjoyable and soothing; see Tips)

15 drops sweet orange essential oil (or any essential oil you find enjoyable and soothing; see Tips)

Clean and dry a 4-ounce (120-ml) bottle. You can buy a new one or repurpose one you already have. I like using a spray bottle; I find it so easy to spritz out the oil into the palm of my hand, rather than carefully pouring. But any type of bottle will work.

Pour the rose-infused jojoba oil into the bottle. Add the lavender and sweet orange essential oils. Swirl the bottle to blend the oils and allow 24 to 48 hours for the scent to settle and develop.

To use, massage about 1 teaspoon or about 5 spritzes of oil all over your body. Breathe in the aroma and have yourself a good night!

TIPS: Pour a little of this blend into a rollerball bottle, and use anytime you want to bring feelings of relaxation and calm to your day!

Other soothing oils used for relaxation are spruce, cedarwood, bergamot, rose, clary sage, frankincense, vanilla and geranium. I personally love the blend of 5 drops each of cedarwood, geranium and sweet orange.

Body Butter

Body butters are all about feel-good indulgence. Our skin is a sense organ, which means the experience that skin care provides on the outside can make a big difference in the way you feel on the inside! Here, solid butters are whipped into an airy, pillowy, gratifying texture that feels like being wrapped in the coziest blanket!

I hope you give this recipe a go! I've made body butters a million different ways, and this "no-melt" version is the simplest to make yet produces the best, creamiest result.

Skin type: all skin types | ***Shelf life:*** 6 months

½ cup (114 g) shea butter

⅓ cup (72 g) mango butter

3½ tbsp (53 ml) jojoba oil

30 drops essential oil of choice (see Tips)

In a large bowl, add the shea and mango butters. Blend with a handheld blender and then drizzle in the jojoba oil. Add the essential oil and continue blending for 5 minutes.

Put the butter in a widemouthed jar. You can also pipe it into your jar if you want to have a buttercream-like swirl at the top.

To use, scoop out a small dollop of body butter and apply it all over, especially on any areas that need extra moisturizing attention. It's best to apply the body butter onto damp skin, right after a shower. It will absorb very quickly and leave you feeling soft and smooth!

TIPS: The ratio used in this recipe is 50 percent shea butter, 30 percent mango butter and 20 percent jojoba oil. You can use that ratio to make any amount you'd like.

My favorite blend of essential oils is 25 drops of grapefruit essential oil and 5 drops of ylang ylang essential oil; it smells fresh, bright and a little floral.

Use an Herbal-Infused Oil (pages 18–19), like that used in the Chai Tea Scrub (page 110), to bring added benefits and aroma!

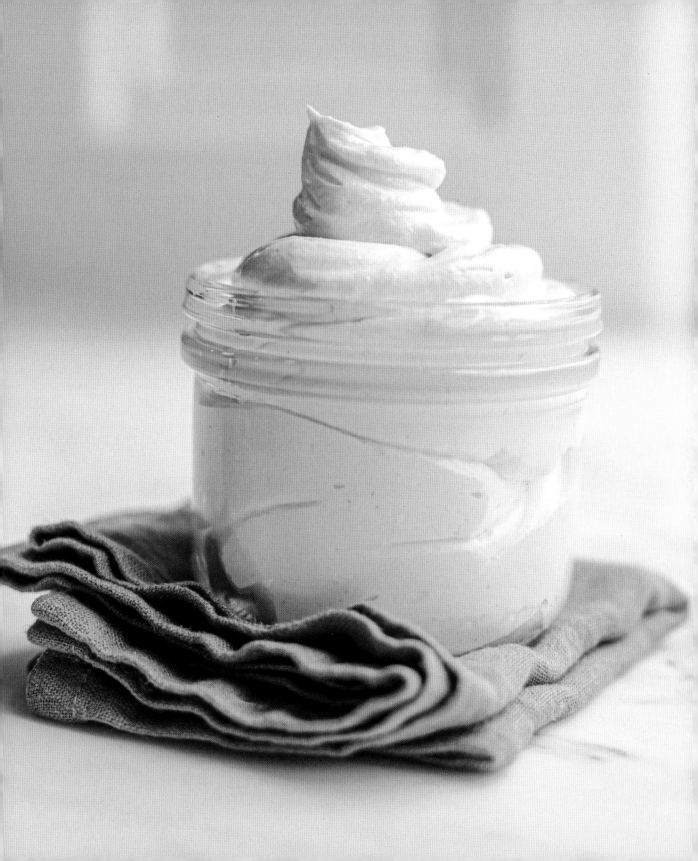

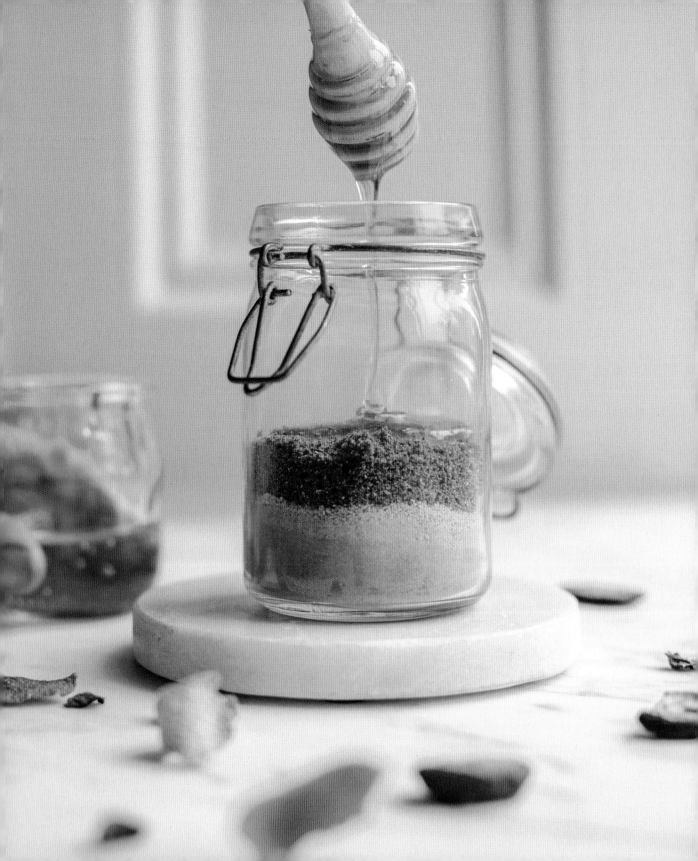

Masks

Masks are a healthy diet for the skin. They sit on the skin, so that the ingredients can penetrate deeply. Masks are the best way to deliver a feast of concentrated nutrient-dense nourishment. Masks also strengthen the functions of the skin.

Make masks a part of your shower routine, applying a mask right before you step into the shower. The warmth of the steamy air will actually help the ingredients penetrate deeper. Then, at the end of your shower, under the stream of water, you can wash it off easily and mess free.

The difference this daily practice creates for you and your skin might just make it your favorite part of your wellness routine! I hope you enjoy the simplicity of these recipes. It's not necessary to overcomplicate things—healthy skin can truly be this simple.

Here are a few tips about creating your own masks:

Shelf life: To make using a mask easier and more practical, most of the recipes in this book are made of dry powders, which means you can make a big batch and it will last for 3 months. You don't need to mash and blend fresh masks every day or worry about spoilage. The moment you combine the dry mask powders with water or fresh ingredients, the mask comes to life, becomes active and is ready to use right away.

Essential oils: You can add essential oils to the powder and honey mask recipes. The formula is 1 percent dilution, or 1 drop of essential oil for every 1 teaspoon of product. This means you should measure out the total amount of teaspoons going into the recipe you're making, then add the correct amount of essential oil drops directly into the powder or the honey.

Activation: Sprinkle the mask powder into a small bowl, add droplets of water or milk and mix to form a creamy mask consistency. I use a teaspoon to mix the mask and the back of the spoon to apply it to my skin.

Usage: Use clay masks only once per week, or if you are clearing acne, you can use clay masks as a weeklong protocol (use the clay mask daily for one week only). All other masks in this book can be used daily.

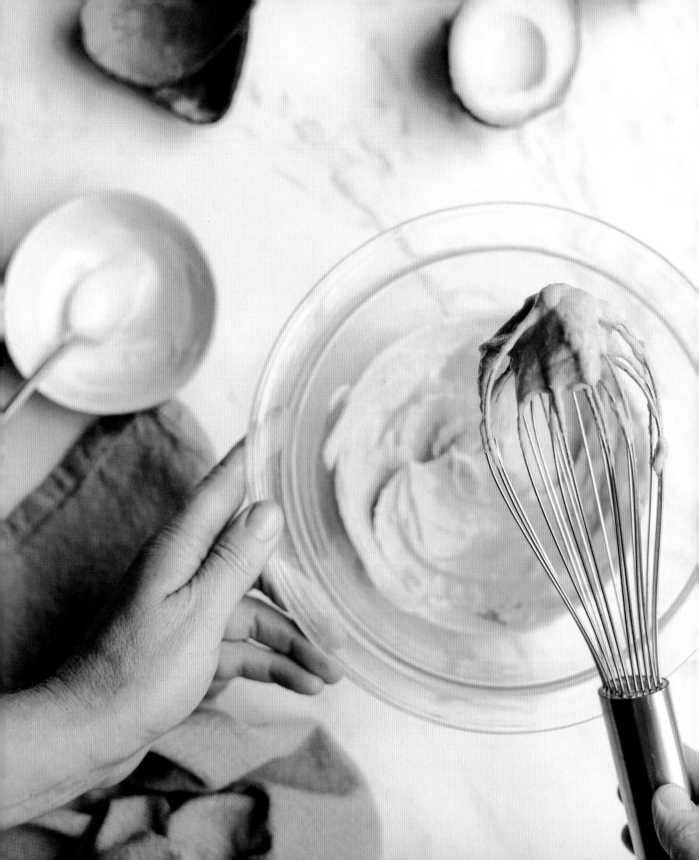

Avocado Purée Moisture Pack

Full disclosure: most days I'd rather eat my avocado than wear it, but if you do slice open an avocado and find that it's not as perfect as you'd like, don't feel frustrated! Turn it into a soothing and moisturizing mask opportunity. Let the delicious fatty acids replenish your skin, leaving it incredibly soft and supple. With a touch of oats to soothe and yogurt to effortlessly dissolve dead skin cells, you'll be left feeling smooth, moisturized and happy!

Skin type: all skin types, especially dry skin | ***Shelf life:*** 1 day

---

1 avocado

1 tbsp (20 g) yogurt

1 tbsp (6 g) oat powder (see Information about Ingredients, pages 147–148)

3 tbsp (45 ml) boiling water

The secret to a great fresh-food mask is working it into a silky-smooth texture. You don't want chunks of avocado on your face! If you only use a fork to mash it, chances are it will be chunky and end up clogging the sink, so I recommend using a blender to make this recipe.

Scoop out the fresh avocado and blend it with the yogurt in a bullet blender or with a small handheld blender until it becomes smooth, like a purée. Set it aside.

Add the oat powder to a large bowl and drizzle in the boiling water, stirring until it forms a creamy oatmeal texture. What we want to collect is just the oat milk and the mucilage—that's where the medicine is. Put the oatmeal through a fine-mesh sieve over a small bowl, straining out the oats and collecting the rich, thick cream in the bowl. Discard the oats.

In the blender or using a handheld blender, blend the avocado-yogurt purée with the creamy oat milk you collected in the bowl. Mix this up well and then apply it to your skin. Let it sit for at least 15 minutes before washing off.

This recipe makes a large amount of product; the idea is to use up an avocado that you may have ended up throwing out. You can always cut the recipe and make a smaller amount, or better yet, wear this mask on your skin and your hair as well!

TIPS: Putting care into the details of all the steps of this recipe will make the difference between a frustrating and a gratifying experience with your mask! Blend the avocado–yogurt and strain the oats well for the best results.

This fresh mask can be used as a deep moisturizing hair treatment, too. Apply it to your hair all the way down to the ends.

Super Greens Powder Mask

If you have powdered greens in your kitchen, you have the makings of amazing skin care! Superfood green powders are made of dehydrated and powdered vegetables and fruits. This mask recipe is all about nourishing the skin. The color alone of a green powder tells you about the density of nutrients that go into this mask. That vibrant green indicates it's incredibly high in chlorophyll, the substance that feeds plants energy from the sunlight. On skin, chlorophyll has a protective and anti-inflammatory effect, but it is also very purifying and cleansing, releasing toxins in the skin. This mask is good for all skin types to build health and resiliency in the skin, but acne-prone skin especially will benefit from "wearing" greens.

Skin type: all skin types, especially acne-prone or dull skin | ***Shelf life:*** 3 months in powdered form, 1 day when activated with water

---

4 tbsp (32 g) greens powder blend

4 tbsp (20 g) kaolin clay

4 tbsp (32 g) coconut milk powder

Clean and dry a jar for storing the mask powder. Fill the jar with the greens powder, kaolin clay and coconut milk powder. Depending on the size of the jar and amount you want to make, you can easily adjust the measurements, filling the jar with one part of each ingredient. Instead of coconut milk powder, you can also use the milk powder of your choice—buttermilk, cow's milk or goat milk. They all deliver fatty moisture to the skin.

To use, scoop out 1 tablespoon (10 g) of the powdered mask mixture into a small bowl. Drizzle droplets of water over the powder and stir to activate the mask, adding enough water to achieve a creamy consistency. Apply the mask to your skin and allow it to sit for 15 minutes. Remove with a soft cotton cloth and water.

TIP: If you don't have powdered milk, use just the greens powder and kaolin clay for your dry mixture and add fresh cow's milk or coconut milk to activate the mask instead of using water.

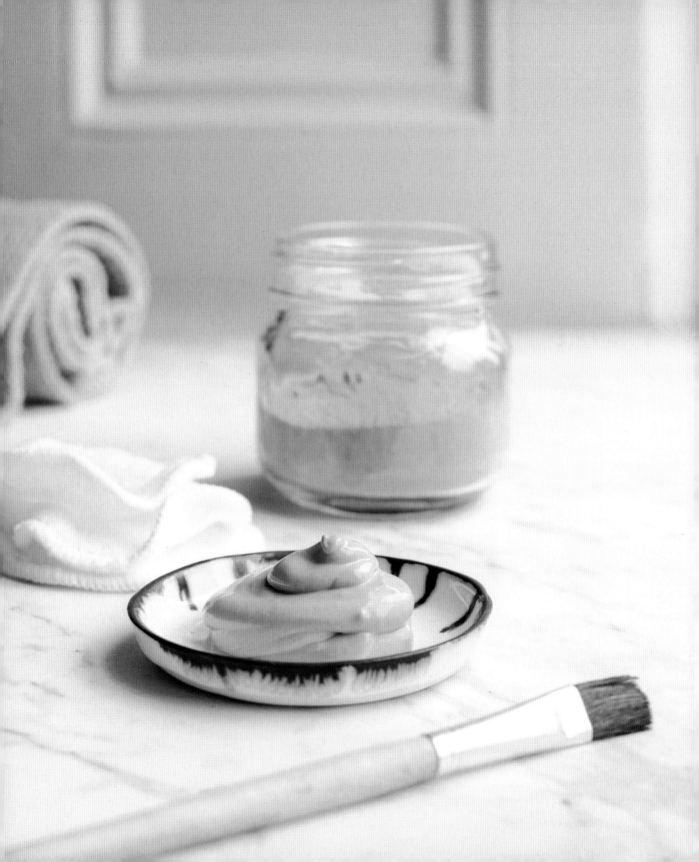

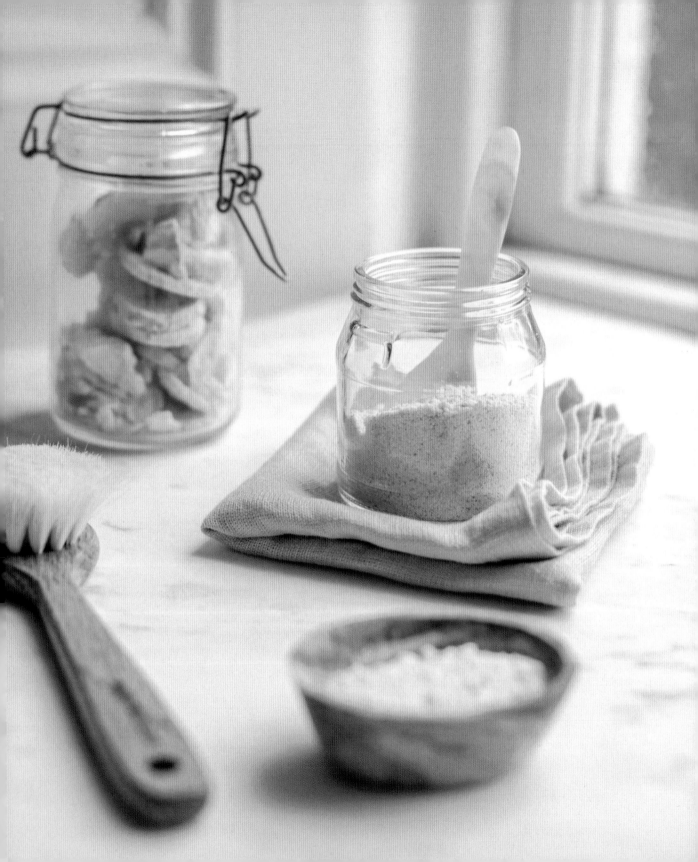

Moisturizing Banana Powder Mask

This mask formulation gives you the moisturizing benefits of creamy fresh bananas but with the convenience of a powdered blend. Freeze-dried bananas deliver a ton of moisture and hydration to skin. I know that dry skin can feel so uncomfortable . . . so we're not stopping there! With extra moisturizing oats and coconut milk, this mask will help parched skin feel satisfyingly quenched, plump and happily restored.

Skin type: dry, dehydrated skin | **Shelf life:** 3 months in powdered form, 1 day when activated with water

---

4 tbsp (24 g) freeze-dried banana powder (see Information about Ingredients, pages 147–148)

4 tbsp (32 g) oat powder (see Information about Ingredients, pages 147–148)

4 tbsp (32 g) coconut milk powder

To a dry 8-ounce (240-ml) container with a lid, add the banana powder, oat powder and coconut milk powder. Close the lid and shake well to mix and incorporate the dry ingredients. Label the jar and keep it well sealed, so that the ingredients do not rehydrate or get wet (see Tip).

To use, add 1 tablespoon (10 g) of the powdered mask to a small bowl. Drizzle droplets of water over the powder and stir to activate the mask, adding enough water to achieve a creamy consistency. Apply the mask to your skin and allow it to sit for 15 minutes. Remove with a soft cotton cloth and water. After removing the mask, seal your damp skin with a few drops of Facial Serum (page 71) to lock in all the new moisture and hydration.

TIP: Freeze-dried banana can rehydrate in a humid environment. If your powdered mask begins to clump, store it in the freezer. Because there's no water content, the dried powders do not freeze and will stay bone dry and powdery! Simply scoop out a helping when you are ready to make a mask.

Vitamin C Mask

Vitamin C is an antioxidant for the skin that neutralizes free radicals from environmental damage, brightens the complexion and stimulates the production of collagen. It's no wonder vitamin C is such a popular skin-care ingredient. This mask features vitamin C–rich raspberry, orange and rose—and because vitamin C is water-soluble, we're using honey to extract it and make it available for your skin to soak up.

Skin type: all skin types | **Shelf life** 3–6 months

---

1 tbsp (7 g) freeze-dried raspberry powder (see Information about Ingredients, pages 147–148)

1 tbsp (5 g) orange peel powder (see Information about Ingredients, pages 147–148)

1 tbsp (3 g) rose petal powder (see Information about Ingredients, pages 147–148)

¼–½ cup (60–120 ml) raw, unfiltered honey (the amount you need will depend on the size of the jar you are using and whether the honey is thick or runny)

Clean a widemouthed glass jar. I recommend using a small jar—less than 8 ounces (240 ml)—so that you can get a feel of the mask before making larger amounts.

Add the raspberry, orange peel and rose petal powders to the clean jar; the jar should be about halfway filled with the blend of powders. Pour in the honey, making sure the powders are fully saturated. Mix with a spoon to release air pockets, and continue adding honey until the herbs are fully covered.

Seal the jar, label it and let it sit to infuse for 2 weeks before using. After 2 weeks, you can try to strain out the powder, but I suggest leaving it in. This will give your mask a scrubby feel, providing a perfect exfoliation when you massage it on your skin.

To use, clean off makeup with the Makeup Melt Cleansing Oil (page 17). With your face slightly damp, apply the honey mask. Let it sit for at least 15 minutes. Before you remove the mask, massage your skin with wet fingertips to take advantage of the gentle exfoliation. Remove the mask with a soft cloth and water.

TIP: This mask is actually delicious! Stir a little in your cup of tea or drizzle over a slice of toast—you'll still get the benefits from the inside out!

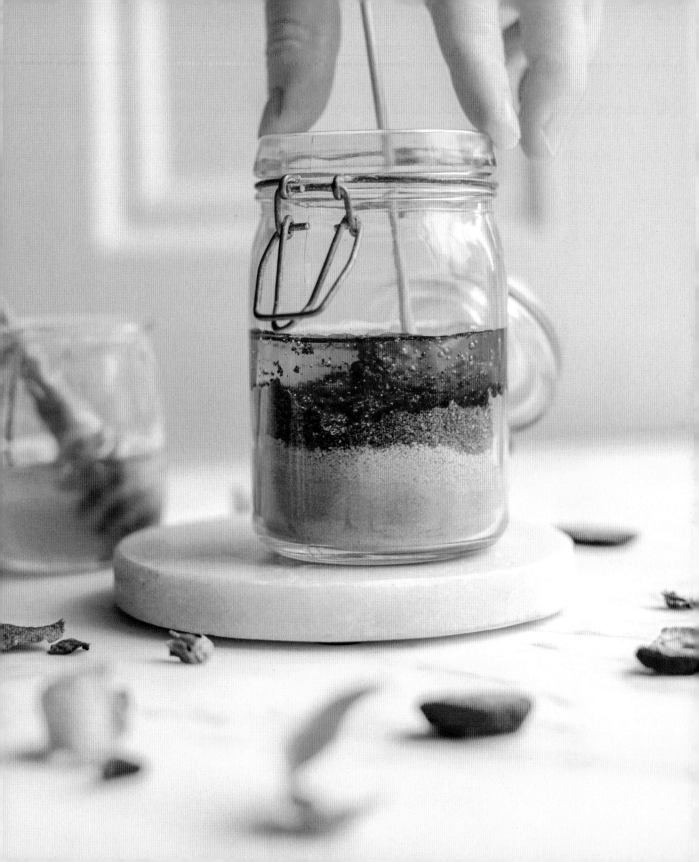

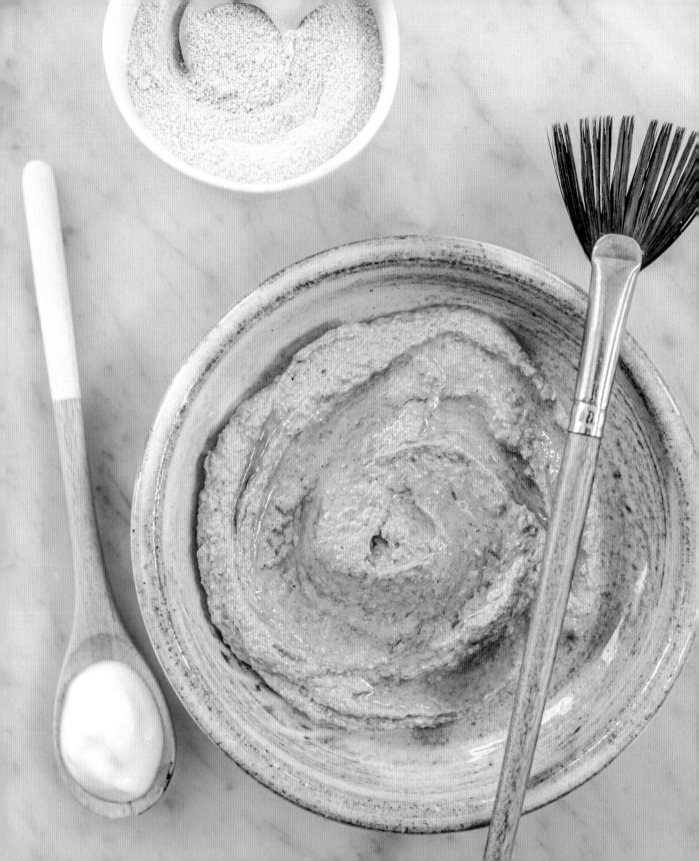

Stress-Relief Mask

Stressed? Inflamed, like all the time? There are herbs for that! Inflammation is the body's response to stress, and stressed-out skin can become red, irritated and sensitive. Using anti-inflammatory herbs can help to soothe the redness and irritation and build resilience in your skin.

This sunshine-yellow mask features two anti-inflammatory superstars—chamomile and turmeric—to give your skin the immediate comfort it needs, so that you can focus your attention on getting to the root of what your inflammation is trying to tell you!

Skin type: all skin types, especially inflamed or acne-prone skin | ***Shelf life:*** 3 months

---

1 tbsp (8 g) oat powder (see Information about Ingredients, pages 147–148)

4 tbsp (8 g) chamomile powder (see Information about Ingredients, pages 147–148)

4 tsp (7 g) kaolin clay

1 tbsp (9 g) turmeric powder (see Tip)

1 tsp full-fat plain yogurt

1 tsp raw, unfiltered honey

In a small blender, bullet blender or spice grinder, add the oat powder, chamomile powder, clay and turmeric powder and process, incorporating all of the ingredients together. Store in a jar, and label and date it!

To use, scoop out 1 tablespoon (8 g) of the powder mixture into a small bowl, and activate it by combining it with the yogurt and honey, mixing well until it reaches a creamy consistency.

Let the mask sit and steep for a couple of minutes, which allows the ingredients to activate and release their precious nutrients. Add a few droplets of water at a time if the mixture becomes too thick. Apply the mask to your face and let it sit for at least 15 minutes. Wash off with water and a soft cloth (be aware that turmeric can stain your cloth yellow; see Tip).

When your skin is inflamed and irritated, it's important to protect it from further stress and irritants, so I recommend following this mask treatment with the Healing Balm (page 68).

TIP: Wash this mask off in the shower, under the stream of water, to avoid a turmeric-stained mess in your bathroom sink. Also, full disclosure: it may temporarily tint your skin, so don't do this mask just before going out! If you're thinking that using the turmeric sounds messy, know that turmeric has been used for the skin for centuries, because it works! It's worth it. The yogurt and honey seem to help prevent turmeric from actually staining the skin. If you do see a yellow tint, the Rice Flour Facial Scrub (page 117) will remove it! If you are really nervous about the yellow color (don't be), search online for "poolan kilangu," which is a white turmeric.

Juice Cleanse Mask

The benefits of fruit for the skin are the natural fruit acids, also known as alpha hydroxy acids. They go to work releasing congestion, resurfacing skin cells and leaving you with a smoother skin texture and brighter complexion. The challenge is making a fruit mask that is shelf stable, so that you don't need to whip up fresh fruit every time you want to use it. Freeze-dried fruit solves that problem!

Skin type: all skin types, especially dry and acne-prone skin | ***Shelf life:*** 3 months

---

2 tbsp (14 g) freeze-dried strawberry powder (see Information about Ingredients, pages 147–148)

2 tbsp (14 g) freeze-dried blueberry powder (see Information about Ingredients, pages 147–148)

2 tbsp (16 g) coconut milk powder

Add the freeze-dried strawberry and blueberry powders and the coconut milk powder to a small blender, bullet blender or spice grinder, and blitz until they are well combined.

Pour the powder into a clean, dry jar; label and date it and seal tightly. I highly recommend that you store this mask powder in the freezer. There it will remain bone-dry, and you won't be worried about the humidity in the air rehydrating the fruit powders.

When you are ready to use the mask, simply scoop out a tablespoon (8 g) of the fruit mask powder and activate by adding a few droplets of water and stirring until the mixture has a creamy consistency. Wear on your skin for 10 minutes and remove with water.

TIP: The coconut milk powder gives the mask a creamier consistency and fatty moisture for the skin. Find coconut milk powder online and store it in the freezer; it's so good to have this ingredient on hand for your skin care.

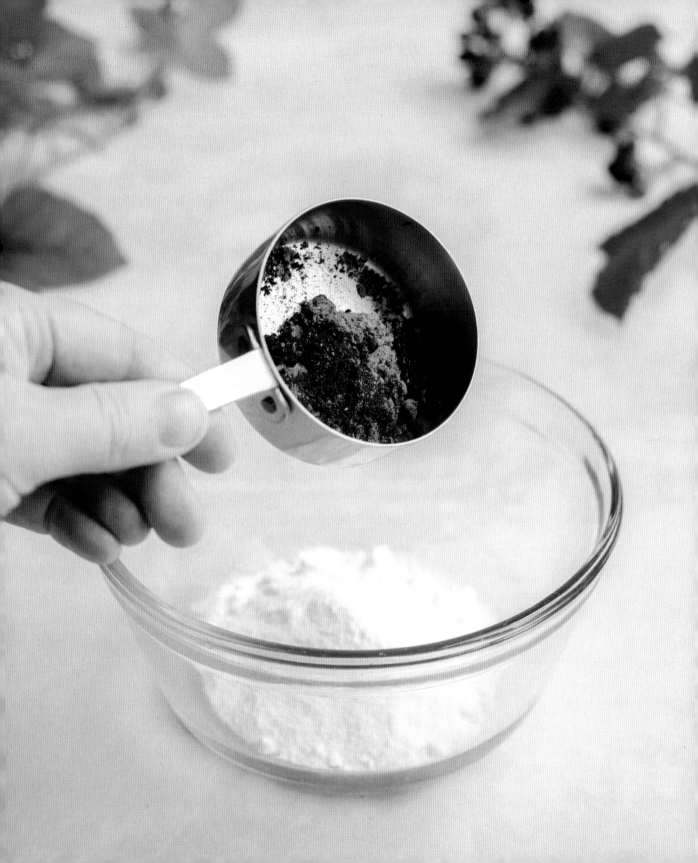

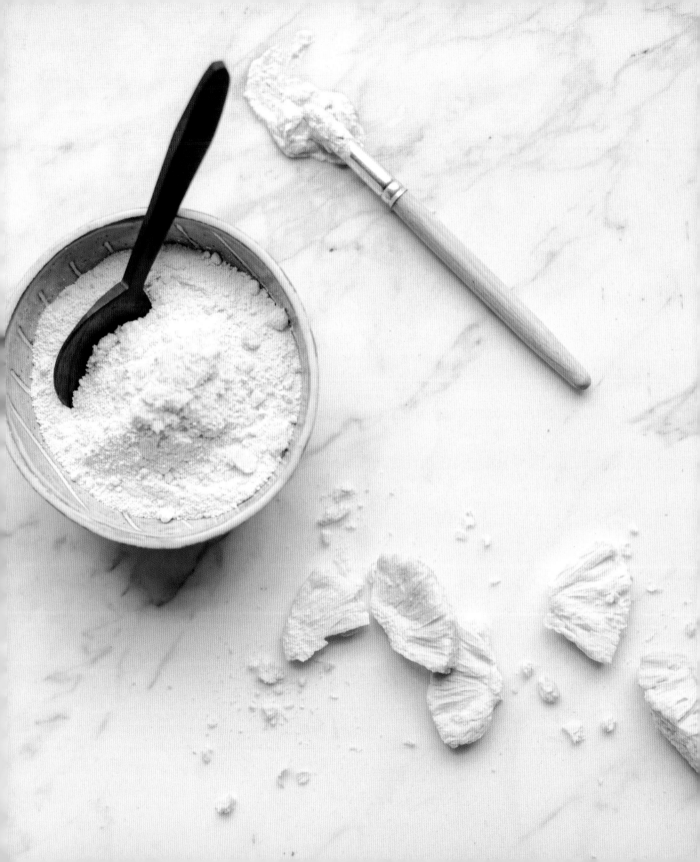

Renew You Mask

This blend is potent! It resurfaces your skin, as if you'd had a professional treatment done. Pineapple is rich in an enzyme called papain, which breaks down the congestion in your skin. Buttermilk is rich in lactic acid, a gentle acid that eats away at dead skin cells. It's also rich in fat, leaving your skin soft and plump.

Skin type: all skin types, especially dry, congested, dehydrated or aging skin |
Shelf life: 3 months

---

1 tbsp (7 g) freeze-dried pineapple powder (see Information about Ingredients, pages 147–148)

4 tbsp (44 g) buttermilk powder

1 tbsp (5 g) kaolin clay

In a small blender, bullet blender or spice grinder, blitz the freeze-dried pineapple powder, buttermilk powder and kaolin clay to mix all of the ingredients together.

Store the mask powder in a jar, being sure to label it. I recommend that you keep this powder blend in the freezer so it doesn't rehydrate. To use, scoop 1 tablespoon (10 g) of the powder into a small bowl. Drizzle droplets of water over the powder and stir to activate the mask, adding enough water to achieve a paste consistency. Wear on your skin for 10 minutes, then wash off with water.

TIP: This makes an incredible bath soak for your whole body! Blend with a cup (240 g) of Epsom salts and come out totally brand new!

Hydration Mask

In herbalism, there is a class of herbs termed mucilaginous, and they are really exciting for skin care. They swell in water and produce a gel-like consistency. Mucilaginous herbs have been used traditionally to soothe, soften and moisten tissue. There are quite a few in this category, including licorice, slippery elm bark, mullein leaf and marshmallow root.

An easy way to access these herbs is in tea blends! In most supermarkets, you can find good-quality herbal teas in the tea section. Look for a blend called "Throat Remedy"; if you read the ingredients, you'll notice most include mucilaginous herbs!

I'll show you how to turn an herbal tea into a hydrating mask, with a touch of milk to deeply moisturize your skin!

Skin type: dry, dehydrated, inflamed skin | ***Shelf life:*** 3 months

---

6 Throat Remedy tea bags

3 tbsp (24 g) coconut milk powder (see Tips)

3 tbsp (33 g) buttermilk powder (see Tips)

1-2 drops oil or Facial Serum (page 71), optional

Tear open the tea bags and pour the herbs into a small blender, bullet blender or spice grinder. Blitz to turn the tea into powder. Add the coconut milk and buttermilk powders, and blitz again to combine all of the ingredients.

To use, scoop out 1 tablespoon (10 g) of powder and add it to a small bowl. Drizzle droplets of water over the powder and stir to activate the mask, adding enough water to form a creamy paste. You can also add one or two drops of oil or your own Facial Serum (page 71) for extra moisture for your skin. Apply the mask to your skin and let it sit for 15 minutes, then remove with a dampened washcloth. I always prefer to remove my masks in the shower, so that it doesn't make a mess!

TIPS: Make sure you purchase a tea made only with herbs, with no flavoring or additives. There are quite a few good brands on the market. I recommend Traditional Medicinals and Yogi Tea.

Find coconut milk powder online, and store it in the freezer to increase the shelf life. You can replace either the coconut milk powder or buttermilk powder with oat powder in equal amounts.

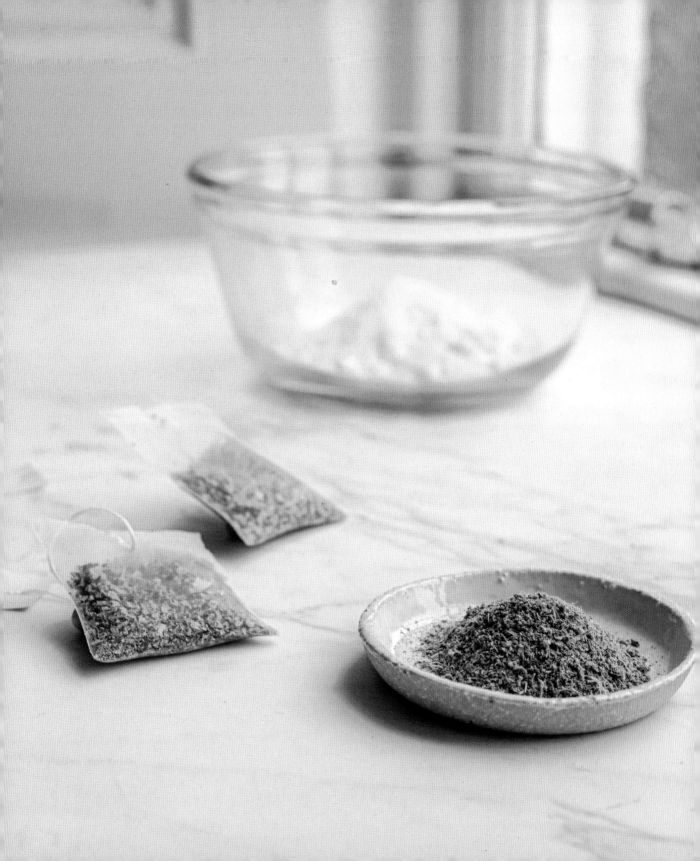

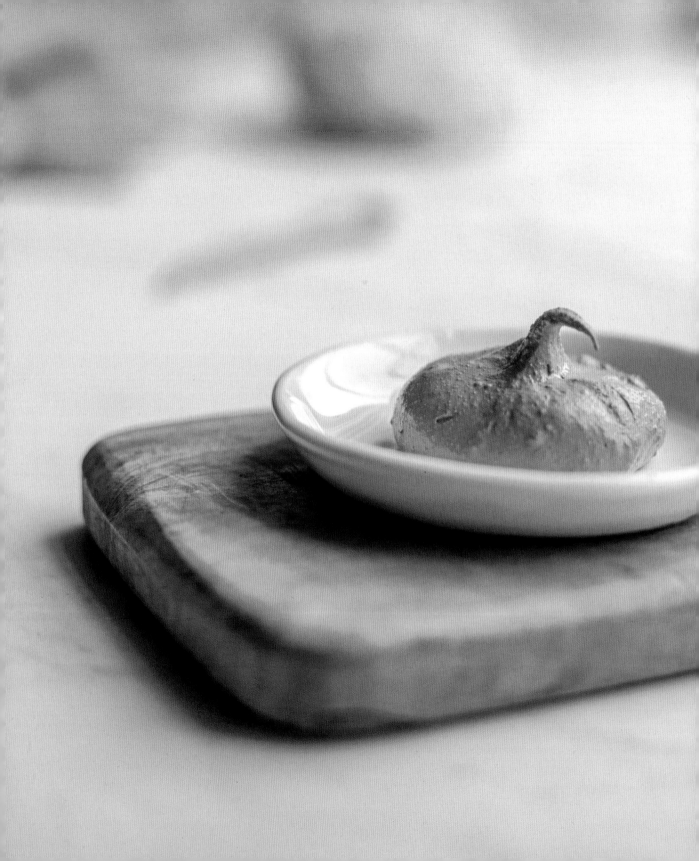

Modern Stress Face Mask

City dwellers, commuters, basically anyone living in an urban environment or working in a large office environment: This mask is for you! Your skin is exposed to an alarming amount of pollution every day—toxins and irritants that can build up and overwhelm the skin. The fumes from cars, smog and poor air quality coupled with the daily grind of modern life begins to stress the body, and it shows up on the skin in the form of inflammation.

As a remedy to the stresses of modern-day life, mushroom tonics, made of powdered medicinal mushrooms, have become incredibly popular. You can find mushroom powder at most health-food stores. Some popular brands are Four Sigmatic, Anima Mundi Herbals and Sun Potion.

Mushrooms are considered adaptogens; they help ease the body's response to stress, boost immunity and reduce inflammation. They are supercharged with anti-inflammatory and antioxidant properties that can help clear acne and eczema and defend the skin against damage. For this remedy, we're using superfood mushroom powder as a superfood face mask! A touch of cocoa powder brings another boost of antioxidants, and kaolin clay deep cleanses. Your skin will stay happy, clean and clear, no matter what's going on around you!

Skin type: all skin types, especially overwhelmed, inflamed or acne-prone skin |
Shelf life: 3–6 months

---

4 tbsp (20 g) mushroom powder
4 tbsp (20 g) cocoa powder
4 tbsp (20 g) kaolin clay

To a widemouthed glass container, add the mushroom powder, cocoa powder and kaolin. Close the lid and shake well to incorporate. When you're ready to use the mask, clean your skin with the Makeup Melt Cleansing Oil (page 17)—even if you're not wearing makeup—to clear away a lot of impurities on your skin. Scoop 1 tablespoon (5 g) of the powdered mask into a bowl and drizzle droplets of water over the powder; then stir to activate the mask, adding enough water to form a creamy paste. Apply the mask to your skin and wear for 15 minutes. I recommend washing this mask off in the shower to avoid a 'shroomy mess on your bathroom counter!

TIP: If you see a mushroom tonic (powder) made with other whole food ingredients like cocoa powder or cinnamon, as long as the additives are herbs or natural ingredients and not an artificial flavoring, you can use it on your skin!

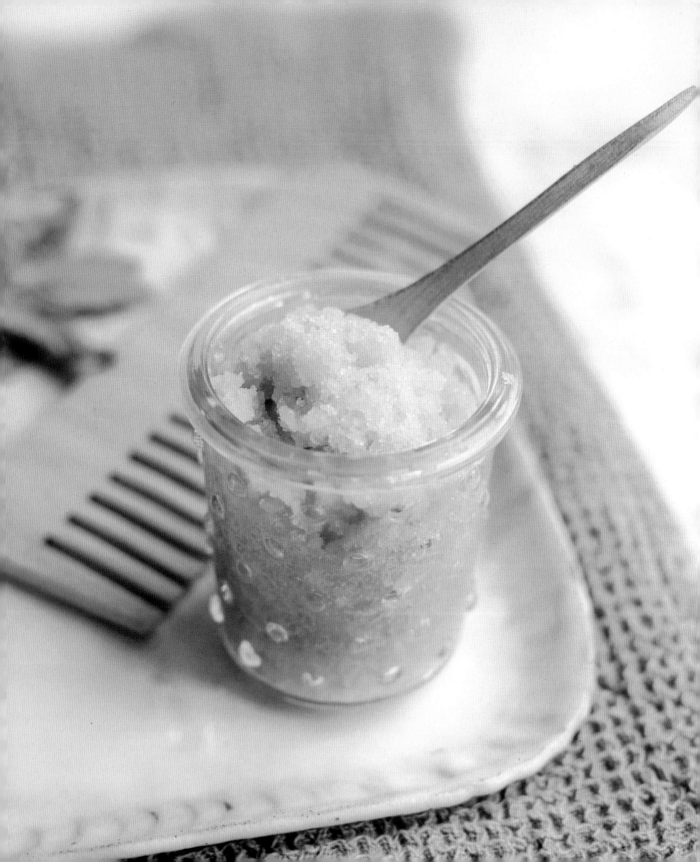

Scrubs

Scrubs are more than surface skin care; I see them as providing full-body wellness. The action of scrubbing activates the lymphatic system to detoxify, stimulate circulation and promote cell turnover. I think scrubs are the best remedy for dryness, stagnation and congestion in the skin. You can feel and see the difference in the texture of your skin after just one use!

Scrubs are made with oil and an exfoliant, usually sugar or salt. I find that most store-bought scrub products are made with grains that are too rough for the skin. After years of experimenting, the recipes that follow make what I think are the best scrubs! By adding my secret ingredients—milk powder and oat powder—these scrubs are very different from what you may be used to! They have a richness to them and melt onto your skin like cream. It's the most enjoyable experience; as you scrub and invigorate your body, you'll feel buttery soft!

Bliss Ball Scrubs (page 122) are transformative—I love making them for friends. The Rose Latte Scrub (page 109) with coconut milk makes your skin feel silky smooth. The Clarifying Scalp Scrub (page 114) even helps your hair grow long and healthy!

You can keep your scrubs in the shower in a tightly sealed container so it doesn't get wet. But make sure to choose a plastic container, because glass can break in the shower (trust me, I speak from experience!).

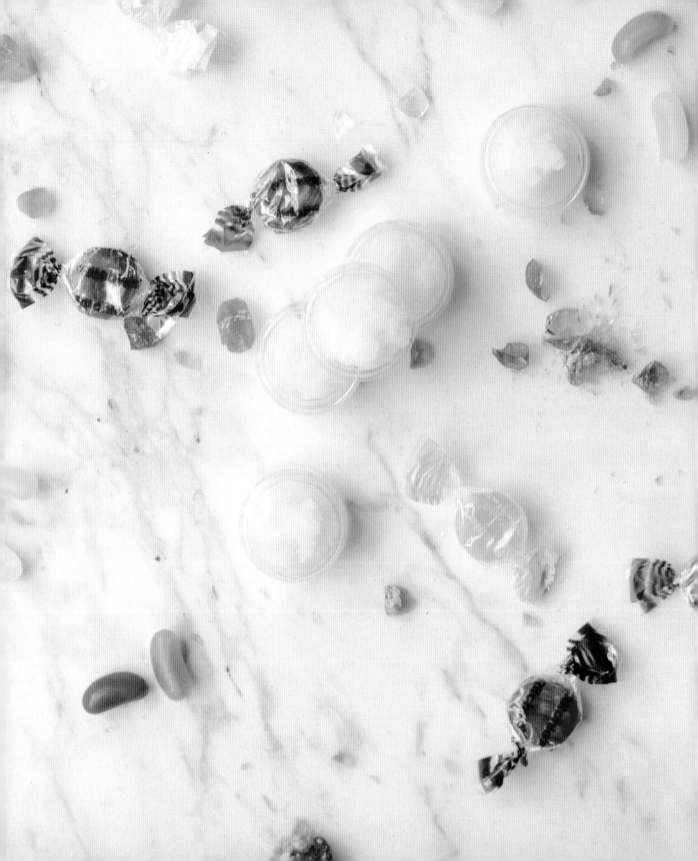

Candy Lip Scrub

This recipe makes the most delicious scrub that you'll ever try! It's fun to use and leaves dry lips feeling plump and smooth. The scent and flavor come from candy flavorings so it's completely edible (and delicious), and when you're finished scrubbing, you get to lick it right off!

Skin type: all skin types | ***Shelf life:*** 3 months

¼ cup (50 g) fine white sugar (see Tips)

2 tbsp (30 ml) jojoba oil (see Tips)

Candy flavoring oil of your choice (see Information about Ingredients, pages 147–148)

Add the sugar to a small blender, bullet blender or spice grinder, and blitz for just a second or two to break down the grains to a finer texture. Pour the sugar into a large bowl. Drizzle in the jojoba oil, mixing well until it reaches a consistency that you like. Some people like a drier scrub, some like a wetter scrub, and there is no right or wrong. Experiment to find the texture you like best.

Add the flavoring oil to taste. You can divide the scrub mixture up and make different flavors. Pot the scrub into small tin containers (see Tips).

To use, scrub your lips gently, enjoying the exfoliation. When you're done, brush off the scrub—or lick it off!

TIPS: Candy Lip Scrubs make great gifts, and making them is a fun party activity for all ages. My daughter makes them with her friends, and they're always a big hit!

Instead of white sugar, you can also use fine brown sugar, which has a different flavor to it. I recommend that you match it with complementary candy flavoring oil, such as chocolate, coffee or pumpkin spice.

In place of jojoba oil, you can choose another neutral oil like sunflower oil or instead go for a more flavorful oil like coconut oil, which pairs well with tropical flavorings, like pineapple or lime.

You can buy tin containers online or in health-food stores, often in the beauty section. Or repurpose an old lip scrub container.

French Vanilla Coffee Scrub

If you respond to the smell of fresh-brewed coffee with enthusiasm, then this scrub will make you feel equally enthusiastic! Coffee acts as a stimulant, and it's become a popular skin-care ingredient for the way it perks up tired skin. But what I've noticed is that too many coffee scrubs are made with rough coffee grains. Even a finely ground coffee can be too scratchy! In this recipe, we blitz the coffee to a powder in the blender, and the result is a scrub that feels smooth and gratifying, just like that first cup in the morning!

Skin type: all skin types | ***Shelf life:*** 3 months

---

3 tbsp (45 ml) coffee-infused sunflower oil (see Herbal-Infused Oil 101, pages 18–19)

2 tbsp (11 g) coffee grounds

2 tbsp (16 g) oat powder (see Information about Ingredients, pages 147–148)

1 cup (200 g) white sugar

1 tbsp (15 ml) vanilla extract

Using coffee-infused oil adds a noticeable boost to the aroma and stimulating benefits of this scrub! Make the infusion (see Herbal-Infused Oil 101 on pages 18–19) over a gentle heat to have it ready in just 6 hours.

In small blender, bullet blender or spice grinder, blitz the coffee grounds into a fine powder. Add the oat powder and sugar, and blitz it for a few seconds to make it finer, but not quite powdered sugar.

To a large bowl, add the powdered ingredients. Begin to drizzle in the coffee-infused oil until the scrub reaches the consistency that you prefer. I personally prefer a drier scrub that resembles wet sand, so that my skin feels soft, but not oily. Add in the vanilla extract and blend well.

Store the scrub in a jar with a lid. Make sure to label and date it. To use, wet your skin in the shower and then turn off the water. Scoop out a generous helping and scrub your body neck to toe. To complement the stimulating effect of the blend and promote circulation, scrub your body in circular motions, always moving toward your heart. For example, start at your ankles and move up your legs, then at your wrists moving up your arms. Go from your neck down your chest and all around your abdomen. Rinse off with water, but do not use soap to wash off the oils—let them soak into your skin.

I recommend doing this scrub in your morning shower! It will wake you up!

TIP: Use flavored coffee grounds—such as pumpkin spice, caramel or peppermint mocha—to change up the scents!

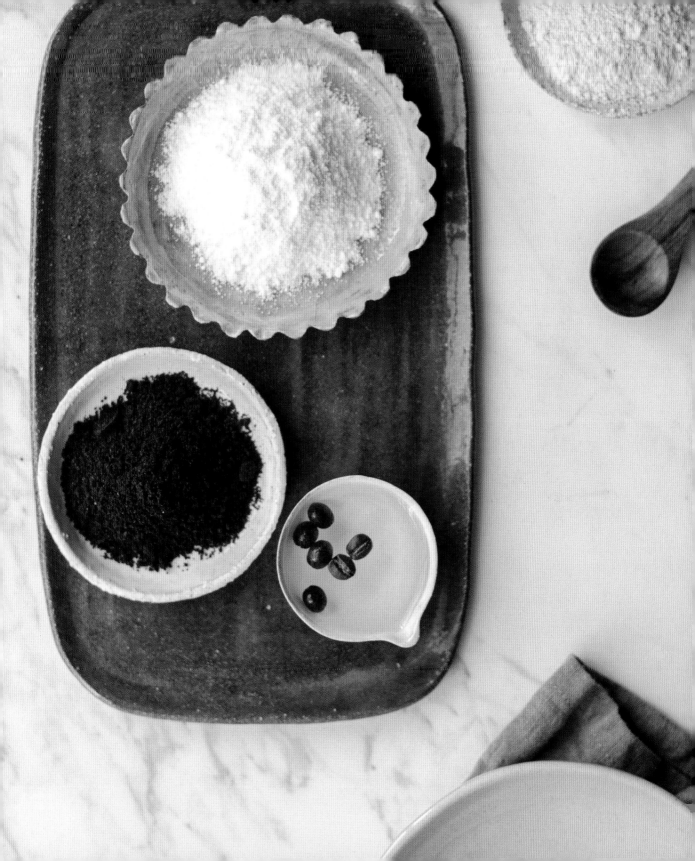

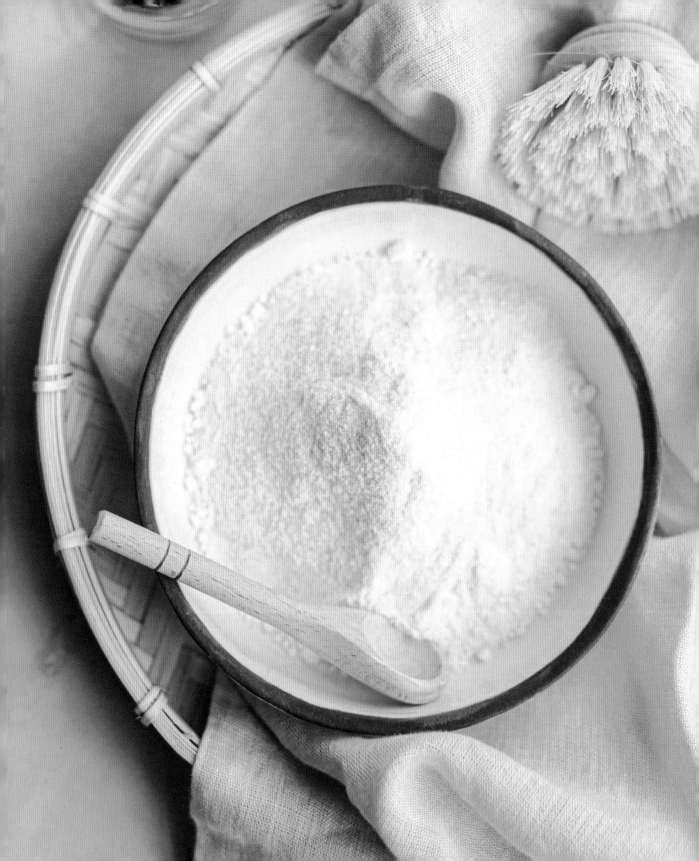

Rose Latte Scrub

The color of this scrub is gorgeous. The soft pink tone comes from Himalayan pink salt, which is very purifying for the skin. With a touch of coconut milk, the scrub feels like silk as it melts over your skin. The entire experience—from the color, to the scent, to the texture—feels incredibly romantic, and this is what I love about skin care. It can create a mood and elevate the way you feel. Make this for yourself and for a loved one.

Skin type: all skin types | **Shelf life:** 3 months

1 cup (300 g) Himalayan pink salt

2 tbsp (16 g) coconut milk powder

3 tbsp (45 ml) rose-infused sunflower oil (see Herbal-Infused Oil 101, pages 18–19)

10 drops rose essential oil or rose-geranium essential oil, optional

In a small blender, bullet blender or spice grinder, blitz the Himalayan pink salt for just a few seconds until the salt is powdery fine. Pour the salt into a large bowl and add the coconut milk powder. Combine well, breaking up any clumps of coconut milk powder. Slowly drizzle in the oil until it reaches the consistency that you like. This recipe is for a "drier" scrub, but you can always add more oil if you like. If you are using essential oils, add them and continue to mix well. Store the scrub in an airtight jar, making sure to label and date it.

To use, step into the shower and wet your skin. Turn off the water and massage a handful of scrub all over. Turn the water back on to rinse, but do not use soap to remove the scrub, as your skin will be clean, soft and moisturized.

TIP: Rose essential oil is very beautiful and also expensive, but never, ever compromise with cheap alternatives. If it's not in your budget, that's okay! Infusing rose petals into oil is a great way to extract the benefits and aroma. Or you can purchase a rose essential oil diluted in jojoba oil. Another option is a natural ingredient called rose wax; search for this online. It's actually the wax from rose petals and is incredibly fragrant. You only need a very small amount—about ⅛ teaspoon—for this recipe. Melt the rose wax with the sunflower oil in a small bowl set in a hot water bath.

Chai Tea Scrub

This scrub features three warming spices: cinnamon, cardamom and ginger. Traditionally these spices have been used topically to help increase blood circulation, which oxygenates the cells, revitalizes skin and brings clarity to the complexion. The warming sensation they bring is also cozy and eases tension. They are excellent for when your muscles are aching and tired. This is a scrub that you'll want to take your time with in the shower. Massage it in slowly and let it sit and soak into the skin—and it will change the way you feel.

Skin type: all skin types | ***Shelf life:*** 3 months

---

1 cup (220 g) brown sugar

1 tbsp (8 g) cinnamon

1 tbsp (5 g) ground ginger

2 tbsp (16 g) oat powder (see Information about Ingredients, pages 147–148)

3 tbsp (45 ml) chai tea-infused sunflower oil (see Tip and Herbal-Infused Oil 101, pages 18–19)

1 tbsp (15 ml) vanilla extract

In a small blender, bullet blender or spice grinder, blitz the brown sugar, cinnamon and ground ginger together, for just a few seconds, to break down the sugar grains and incorporate the spices. Add the sugar mixture to the oat powder. Drizzle in the chai-infused oil, and stir until it forms the consistency that you like. Add in the vanilla extract and mix well.

To use, step into the shower and wet your skin. Turn off the water and scrub all over, neck to toe. Turn the water back on to rinse, but don't wash off with soap—let the fragrant, nourishing and warming oils soak into your skin.

TIP: This recipe calls for chai tea-infused oil, which smells so good! When making your oil, be sure to purchase a chai tea blend that you love the scent of, as this will be the fragrance of your scrub. Save a little for your body oils, body butter or to pour into the bath.

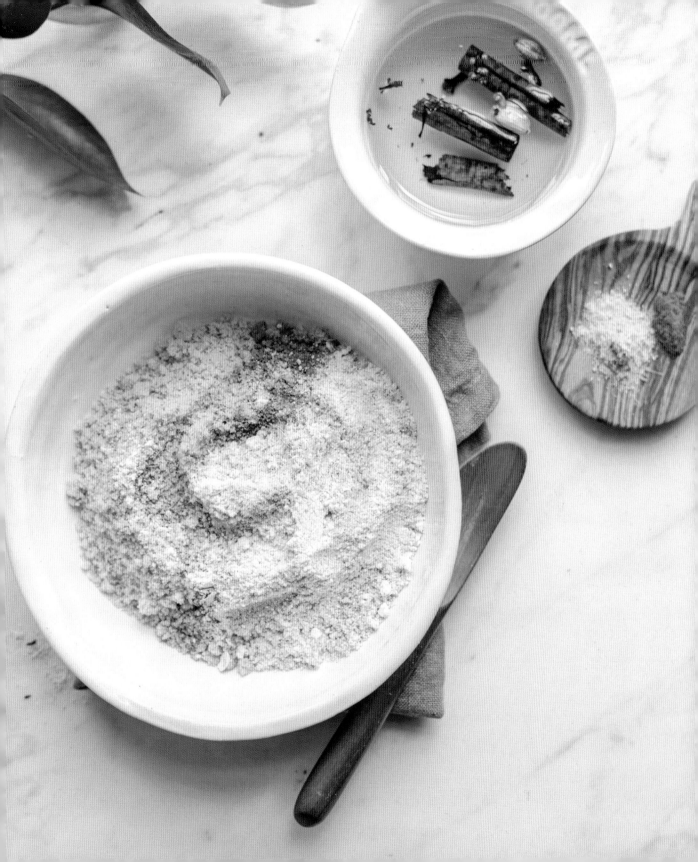

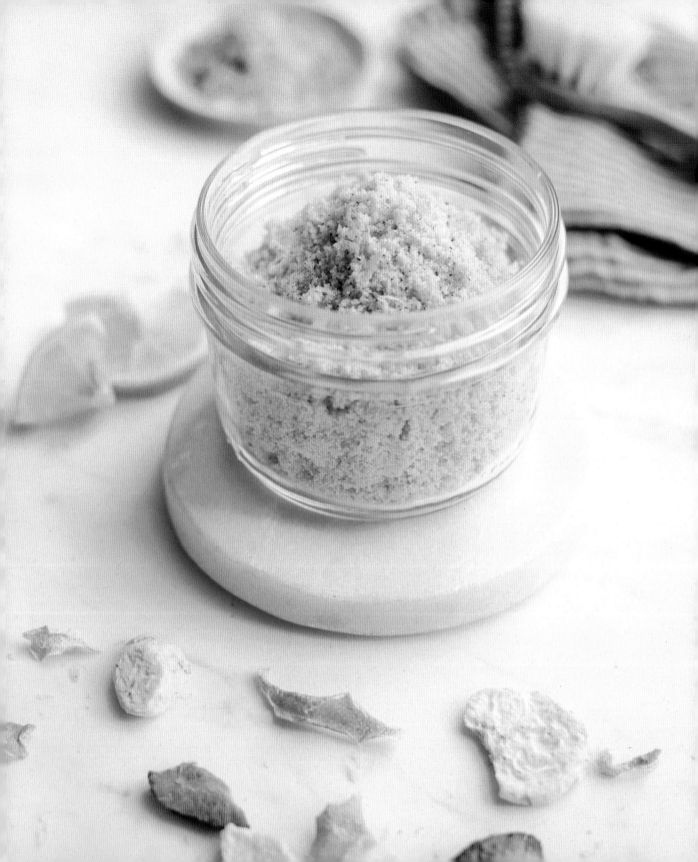

Juice Bar Body Scrub

This fragrant scrub is a sweet, fresh burst of joy for your senses. Alpha hydroxy–rich fruit powders combined with gentle sugar grains leave skin feeling brand new. If you can, leave this scrub on your skin for a few minutes, like a body mask, to let the gentle acids do their resurfacing work.

Skin type: all skin types | **Shelf life:** 1 month

---

1 tbsp (7 g) freeze-dried pineapple powder (see Information about Ingredients, pages 147–148)

1 tbsp (7 g) freeze-dried banana powder (see Information about Ingredients, pages 147–148)

1 tbsp (7 g) freeze-dried strawberry powder (see Information about Ingredients, pages 147–148)

1 cup (200 g) white sugar

2 tbsp (16 g) coconut milk powder

3 tbsp (45 ml) melted coconut oil

Zest of 1 lemon

In a small blender, bullet blender or spice grinder, blitz the freeze-dried pineapple, banana and strawberry powders and the white sugar together until the sugar is ground extra fine, but it is not quite the consistency of powdered sugar. Add the coconut milk powder and blend again until well incorporated.

Pour the powder into a large bowl. Drizzle in the coconut oil and mix until it reaches your desired consistency. Add the lemon zest and mix well.

Store in an airtight jar, making sure to label and date it. To use, step into the shower, wet your skin and turn off the water. Scrub all over. Rinse your skin clean with water, but do not use soap to wash off the oils. Let them soak into your skin.

TIP: This scrub is actually delicious—use it on your lips, too!

Clarifying Scalp Scrub

Healthy hair begins at the roots, yet we often neglect our scalp. Scrubbing your scalp once a week helps to clear away product buildup, release dandruff and stimulate healthy hair growth. This scrub features clarifying sea salt infused with apple cider vinegar, invigorating mint, rosemary and conditioning coconut oil. It leaves your hair, head and mind feeling renewed and refreshed.

Skin type: all skin types | *Shelf life:* 3 months

1 cup (240 ml) apple cider vinegar

¼ cup (7 g) fresh rosemary sprigs

¼ cup (6 g) fresh peppermint leaves

2 cups (285 g) fine sea salt

3 tbsp (45 ml) melted coconut oil

10 drops essential oil, optional (see Tips)

TIPS: If you do not want to go through the process of dehydrating vinegar salt in the oven, simply add a splash of vinegar to the scrub before each use. You can infuse peppermint and rosemary into the vinegar to get the added benefits—follow the Infused Vinegar directions (page 52).

If you want to add scent to this scrub, lavender, rosemary or lemon all work well and add scalp-cleansing properties. You can use combinations of these three scents; use 10 drops of essential oil in total.

In a small blender, bullet blender or spice grinder, blend the apple cider vinegar, rosemary and peppermint for several seconds, until all the herbs are finely ground, turning the vinegar green. Pour the vinegar through a fine-mesh strainer or cheesecloth to separate the herbs. Discard or compost the herbs, reserving the herbal vinegar.

Set the oven to its very lowest setting. If your oven doesn't go below 150°F (65°C), you can leave the door slightly cracked, so that it does not get too hot. In a large bowl, combine the sea salt and the herbal vinegar and then pour it all out onto a baking tray. It's okay if the salt appears to have melted in the liquid. The mixture will have a thick, watery, sludge-like consistency, but it will dehydrate back into salt crystals in the oven.

Put the salt in the oven and keep an eye on it! When the water has evaporated, in 20 to 30 minutes depending on your oven, you will have herbal vinegar salt, which makes the base of this scrub recipe. Remove the salt from the oven and allow it to cool.

In a bowl, combine the infused salt and coconut oil. Mix well to combine. If you are using essential oils to add scent (see Tips), drop them over the mixture and stir well.

To use, wet your hair in the shower. Scoop out a handful of the mixture and begin to scrub your scalp, parting the hair to make sure the product gets on the skin. Close your eyes—you don't want the vinegary salt to run down into them!

Scrub well, rinse thoroughly and follow with shampoo and conditioner as normal. As an experiment, you might skip the shampoo and conditioner to see how your hair responds to this scrub as a natural shampoo alternative!

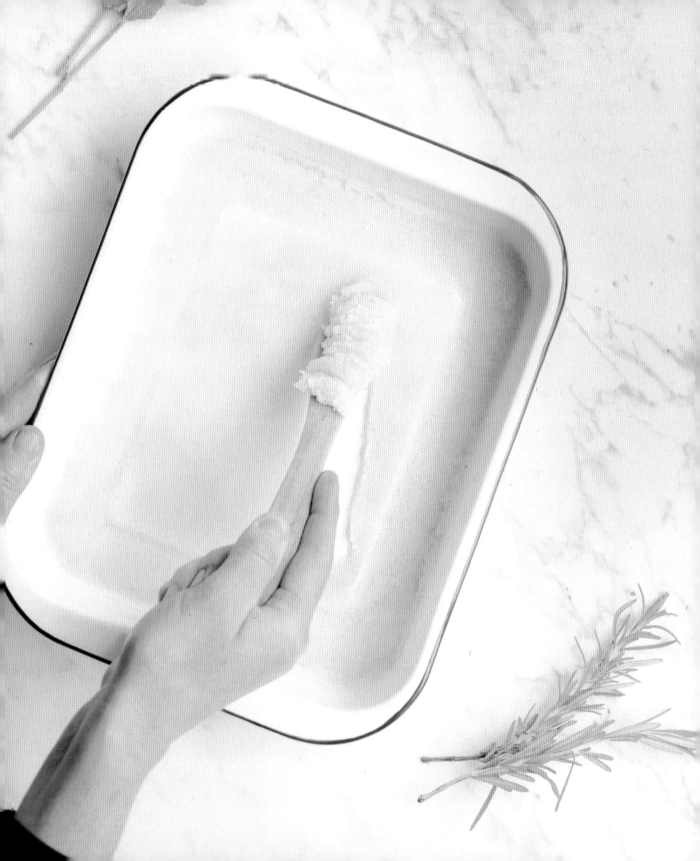

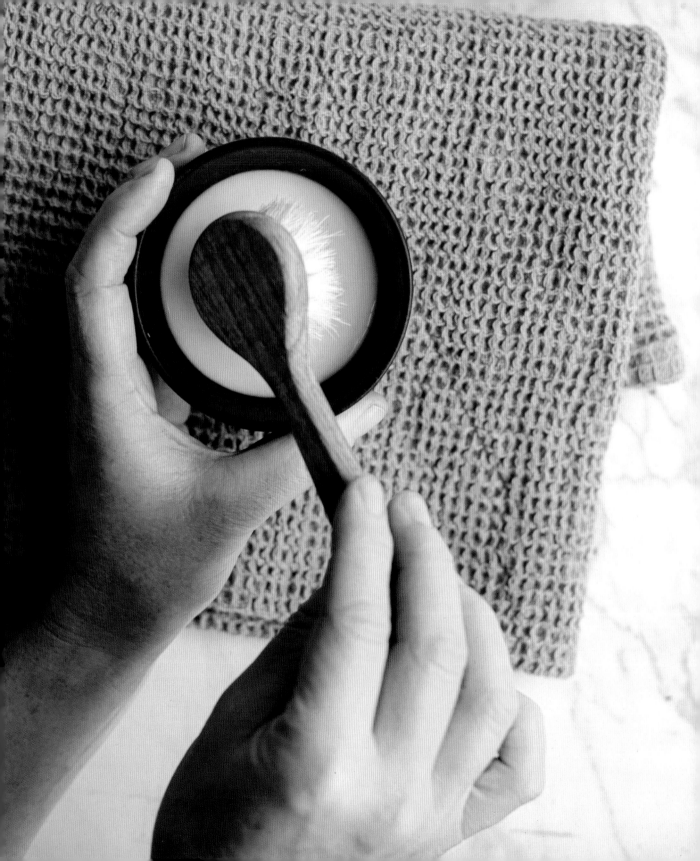

Rice Flour Facial Scrub

This recipe shows off how transformative your own self-made remedies can be for your skin. With one treatment, your skin will feel noticeably smoother and softer! It features a special ingredient, rice flour, which has a texture to it that almost buffs the skin. It's like getting a microdermabrasion treatment at home! It leaves your skin rejuvenated, smooths out texture and brightens your complexion. Don't let the simplicity of this scrub lead you to underestimate its powers! It's very exfoliating, so only do this treatment once per month. Make it fresh each time.

Skin type: all skin types, especially congested, dull, dry skin | ***Shelf life:*** use immediately

2 tbsp (20 g) finely ground white or brown rice flour

1½ tsp (8 ml) jojoba oil

2 tsp (10 ml) water

In a small bowl, combine the rice flour and jojoba oil. The mixture will be thick, but the water will help to thin it out. Drizzle in the water slowly, mixing until the scrub has a creamy consistency.

Clean your skin first with the Makeup Melt Cleansing Oil (page 17). Then begin to gently exfoliate by massaging the scrub all over your face. Do not add pressure with your fingers—be very gentle as the ingredients do all the work. Focus on any areas of your skin that have congestion. Rinse off with water, and follow immediately with your best serum or moisturizer.

TIP: Do not expose your skin to the sun for a few hours after this treatment. I recommend doing this treatment at night.

Creamy Mango Scrub

This recipe features vitamin C–rich mango butter, which is a skin-care favorite because it is a "dry" butter. It soaks in very quickly, with almost a dry finish, leaving your skin feeling supple and soft but never greasy! Combined with the brown sugar crumble and real mango fruit acids, you get an exfoliation treat that you'll love indulging in over and over again!

Skin type: dry skin | **Shelf life:** 3 months

1⅔ tbsp (23 g) mango butter

3 tbsp + 1¼ tsp (51 ml) melted coconut oil, divided

1 cup (220 g) brown sugar

2 tbsp (14 g) freeze-dried mango

Zest of 1 lime

In a large bowl, place the mango butter and 1¼ tsp (6 ml) of coconut oil. Whip with a handheld blending stick for 5 minutes, until well combined and creamy.

In a blender, combine the brown sugar and freeze-dried mango. Blend until the mango pieces are broken down finely and combined into the sugar. Pour this mixture into another large bowl. Add the remaining coconut oil and mix well with a spoon. Add the lime zest and mix to combine.

Scoop the exfoliating crumble into a plastic pot and top with the mango buttercream; you can spoon or pipe it into the jar. You can also layer the buttercream and crumble like a parfait, or combine it before adding it to the pot.

To use, scoop out a generous helping of your scrub, making sure to get lots of those exfoliating crumbles with the buttercream. Get into the shower, but don't turn the water on just yet. Massage and scrub over your entire body, from neck to feet. Turn on the water and use a cotton cloth to rinse off and remove the creamy scrub. Do not wash off with soap to keep all the moisturizing ingredients on your skin. By the time you come out of the shower and dry off, all of the mango butter will have soaked in, leaving your skin incredibly smooth and soft, but not greasy at all!

TIP: You can whip the sugar mixture into the body butter to make a scrubby butter!

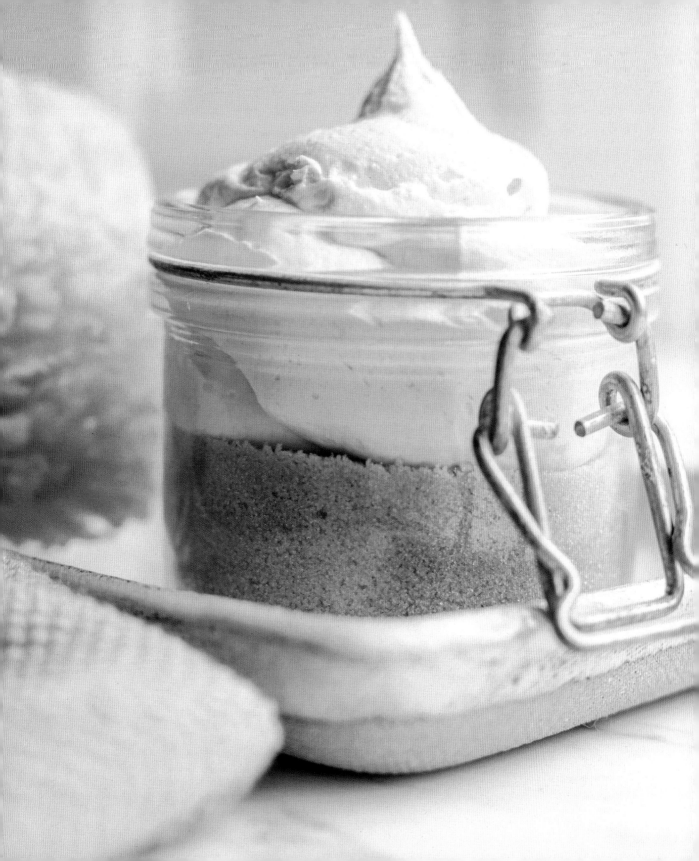

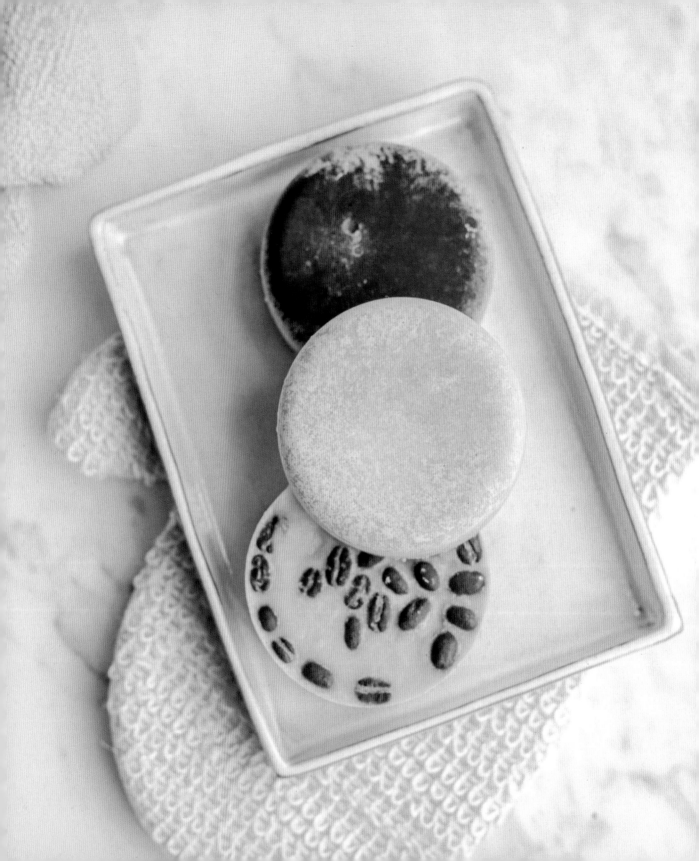

Solid Scrub Bar

This handheld, solid scrub is easy to use in the shower, with no dipping into a jar and no fuss. And further keeping life simple, this one product both deeply moisturizes and exfoliates your skin all at once. Glide this bar all over your body, elbows and feet. I also love exfoliating the parts of the body that we sometimes neglect, such as the underarms, backside and bikini line. The sugar grains remove dead skin cells, and the rich butters melt into the skin, leaving you feeling soft, smooth and comfortable in your skin.

Skin type: all skin types, especially dry skin | ***Shelf life:*** 3-6 months

---

⅓ cup (72 g) cocoa butter, divided

⅓ cup (72 g) shea butter

10–15 drops essential oil of choice, optional (see Tip)

2 cups (400 g) fine white sugar

TIP: I love to use an invigorating blend of 6 drops lavender essential oil and 6 drops peppermint essential oil in my bar, but you can use whatever scent you like. The cocoa butter base gives a light chocolate aroma. It complements well with citrus oils like lime and grapefruit; minty peppermint; floral oils like rose and lavender; and warming oils like ginger, cardamom and vanilla.

Over medium heat, bring a small saucepan of water to a simmer. Set a heatproof bowl over the pot and add half the cocoa butter. Stir continuously, until the cocoa butter is completely melted. Continue stirring, keeping it over the low-simmer heat for another 5 minutes. Then add in the remaining cocoa butter and shea butter, and stir continuously until fully melted. Remove from the heat, and set the bowl on the counter to cool, but not harden. If you are adding in essential oils, add now.

When the melted butters are fully cooled and almost to the point of congealing again, pour in the sugar and mix well. Pour the mixture into molds—I like to use silicone muffin molds. If you do not have molds, use a cake pan, and when fully set, slice the whole block into smaller bars.

Set the molds in the refrigerator to fully harden, about 30 minutes. You can then pop out the bars and store them in an airtight container. During the summer or in a warm environment, the bars can melt. Store them in the refrigerator if that's the case.

To use, bring the scrub bar into the shower. Wet your skin and use the bar to scrub all over. You can keep the bar in the shower but out of direct contact with water so that it doesn't melt. Rinse your skin clean with water and a soft cloth, but do not use soap. Let the butters soak into your skin.

Bliss Ball Scrub

This scrub takes multipurpose all the way. It's a body scrub, cleanser and mask. The balls are dense, but the moment you add water, they will melt into a lush, scrubby cream that you can buff right onto your skin. This recipe features oats, which are rich in saponins and cleanse the skin, with a touch of clay to stimulate and detoxify. Cocoa powder and lavender provide protective and brightening antioxidants that help to fade sunspots.

Skin type: all skin types | **Shelf life:** 3 months

---

2 tbsp (28 g) cocoa butter

1 tbsp (15 ml) oil of choice (coconut, almond, olive, etc.)

¼ cup (32 g) oat powder

1 tbsp (1 g) dried lavender buds

4 tbsp (20 g) cocoa powder, divided (see Tip)

½ cup (145 g) sea salt, or pink Himalayan salt

10 drops lavender essential oil, optional

TIP: Try replacing the cocoa powder with matcha powder or almond flour to create different variations. Cocoa and matcha are both antioxidant-rich, while almond flour is gently exfoliating and moisturizing.

Over medium heat, bring a small saucepan of water to a simmer. Set a heatproof bowl over the pot and add the cocoa butter. As the butter starts to melt, add the oil. Remove the bowl from the heat and set it aside to cool as you prepare the dry ingredients.

In a small blender, bullet blender or spice grinder, blitz the oat powder and lavender buds, and blend until the lavender is finely ground. Pour the ground oats, lavender and 2 tablespoons (10 g) of the cocoa powder through a fine sieve into a large bowl so the mixture is powdery soft and well combined. Blitz the salt for a few seconds in the blender or spice grinder to break down the grains, so that it will be gentler on the skin. Add the salt to the bowl and mix well.

By now, the cocoa butter and oil blend should be cooled down. If you want to add essential oil, stir it into the cooled butter and oil mixture.

Very slowly pour the wet ingredients into the dry ingredients, 1 tablespoon (15 ml) at a time. After each addition, massage and knead the mixture with your hands and continue adding tablespoons of the butter and oil mixture until the mixture has a Play-Doh–like consistency. If you've ever made energy balls, it's almost the same! You may not need to use all the butter and oil mixture to reach this consistency; store any leftovers in a labeled jar for another time.

Roll the dough into balls, and dust them with the remaining 2 tablespoons (10 g) of cocoa powder. Place the balls in the refrigerator for 15 minutes to harden, and then you can keep them in an airtight container in your bathroom cabinet or store in the refrigerator. They travel well and make really fun gifts!

To use, once or twice a week take one ball into the shower. Wet your skin and then turn off the water. I like to break up the ball in the palms of my hands. Massage your skin gently with the ball; the butter will begin to melt as it scrubs. Rinse off the scrub and wipe your skin clean with a soft cloth, but do not use soap; it will clean off the nourishing oils and butters. You can use soap strategically as needed—for example, on underarms or feet—but try to limit the use of soap to just those areas.

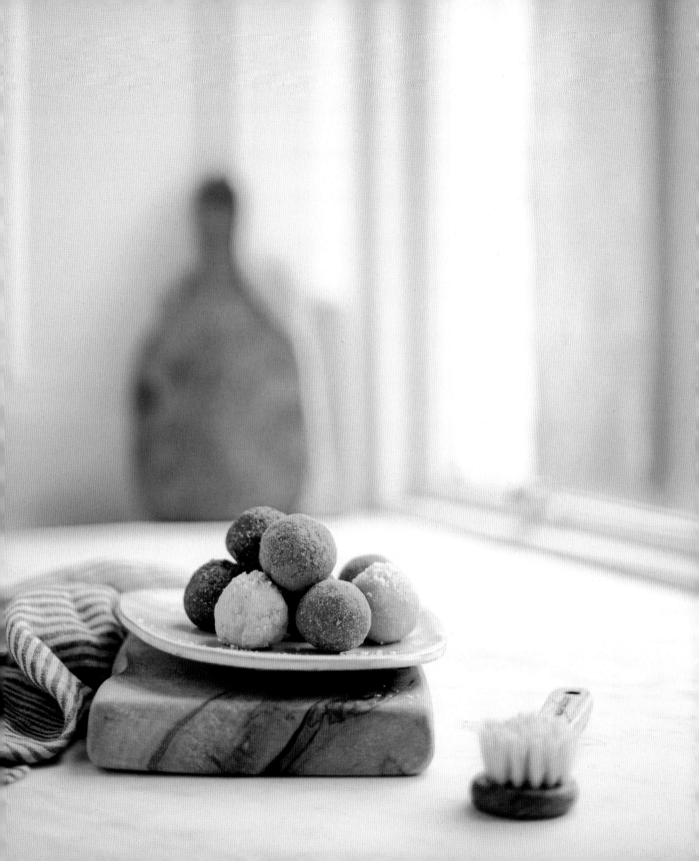

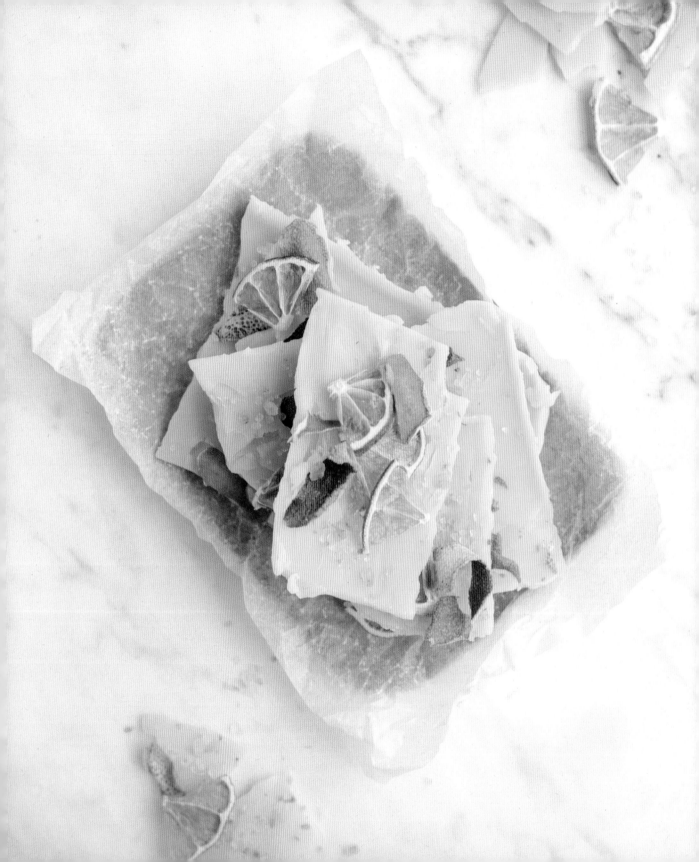

Treats

This chapter celebrates the joy of making skin care. It's playing with beautiful ingredients, getting creative and making something that lights you up and makes you feel good. Food—whether it's what you eat or what you put on your skin—is about nourishment, but it's also about joy. The experience of indulging in the ingredients, the scents and the beautiful colors is part of the beauty that these recipes offer.

This chapter will also help you share these sense experiences with others! I love making the White Chocolate Bath Melt (page 129) and Mylk Bath (page 133) as gifts! You can also make skin care with your friends and family. If you're hosting a party, instead of just having a dessert bar, set up a Bath Tea (page 134) bar with the ingredients for your guests to make their own bath blend. Or, create a fun activity making Flower Cookie Bath Bombs (page 126) together. It can be a fun hands-on experience that all ages will love, and it's a great way to pass along the knowledge and inspiration of making natural skin-care products.

Flower Cookie Bath Bomb

This recipe is for all the bakers out there. The entire process is similar to making cookies, which can be so gratifying! Topped with sugared flowers, making these bath bombs is the perfect way to spend an afternoon in the kitchen, followed by a soak in the tub. Bath bombs are a treat for the senses; they make bath time more enjoyable and fill the bathwater with fragrant botanicals. These treats are fun to make and fun to use!

Skin type: all skin types | ***Shelf life:*** 1–2 months; longer if you seal airtight

---

Sugar Flowers

1 egg white

Assortment of fresh flowers, small enough to fit on a sugar cookie. Look for flowers that lay flat (for example, daisies); you can also use leaves, like sage, mint or lemon balm

¼ cup (50 g) fine white sugar

Bath Bombs

2 cups (440 g) baking soda

1 cup (230 g) citric acid

½ cup (64 g) cornstarch

2 tbsp (22 g) buttermilk powder, optional

2 tsp (10 ml) neutral oil of choice (jojoba, sunflower or grapeseed all work well)

40 drops essential oil of choice (I love 20 drops of sage + 20 drops of grapefruit)

Rubbing alcohol in a spray bottle

To make the sugar flowers, beat the egg white in a small bowl with a whisk or hand blender until frothy. Dip a thin paintbrush into the froth and lightly paint the petals or leaves. Lightly sprinkle the petals or leaves with sugar on both sides, and let them dry overnight. Sugared flowers can be stored in an airtight container; they last forever!

To make the bath bombs, add the baking soda, citric acid, cornstarch and buttermilk powder (if using) to a large bowl. Add the oil and essential oils, and work them through the mixture. I like to use a silicone spatula to smear the oils into the powders. Mix well until all ingredients are well incorporated.

Begin to mist the mixture with rubbing alcohol. You will notice the powders begin to fizz. Keep moving or stirring the mixture with your hands as you mist, so that the powder does not fizz away. Add just a little rubbing alcohol at a time, until the mixture holds its shape when you squeeze it in your hands.

Drop the bath bomb "batter" onto a sheet of parchment paper, and put another sheet of parchment paper on top. Roll the batter flat with a rolling pin to about 1 inch (3 cm) thick. Use a cookie cutter or drinking glass to cut out the cookie shapes. Top with the sugared flowers, gently pressing them into the batter, so that they will stick. Let the cookies sit to dry overnight.

To use, drop one or two into a bath. I like to wait until I'm in the tub to use my bath bomb—it lights me up to see it pop and fizzle in the water! Breathe in deeply as you soak, and enjoy the visual and aromatic experience!

TIP: Make the sugared flowers ahead of time; it's a fun craft activity at home. They store for months in a jar, ready to use when you want them. If you're making these as a group project at a party, either make the sugared flowers in advance, or offer an assortment of dried flowers like rosebuds and lavender.

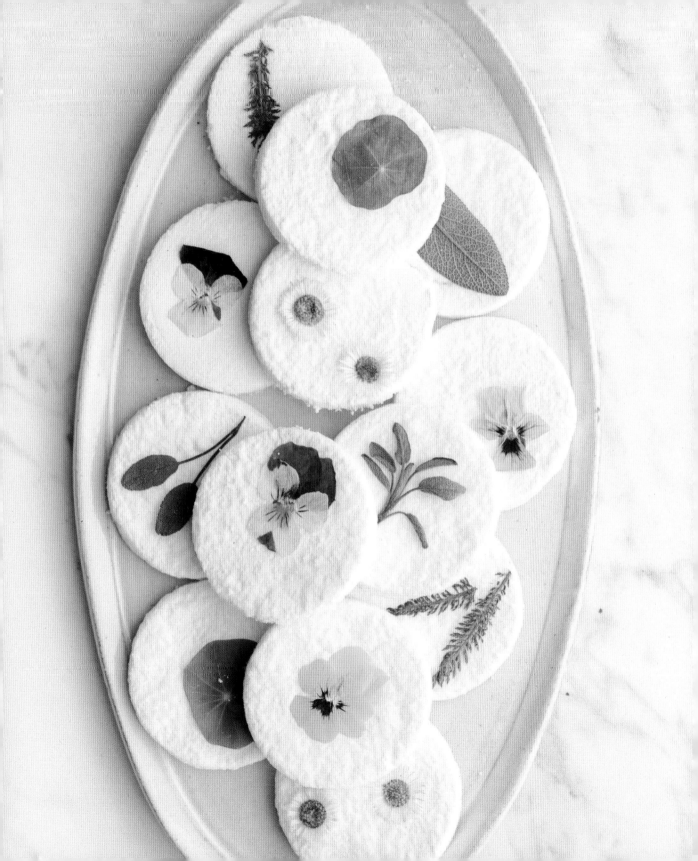

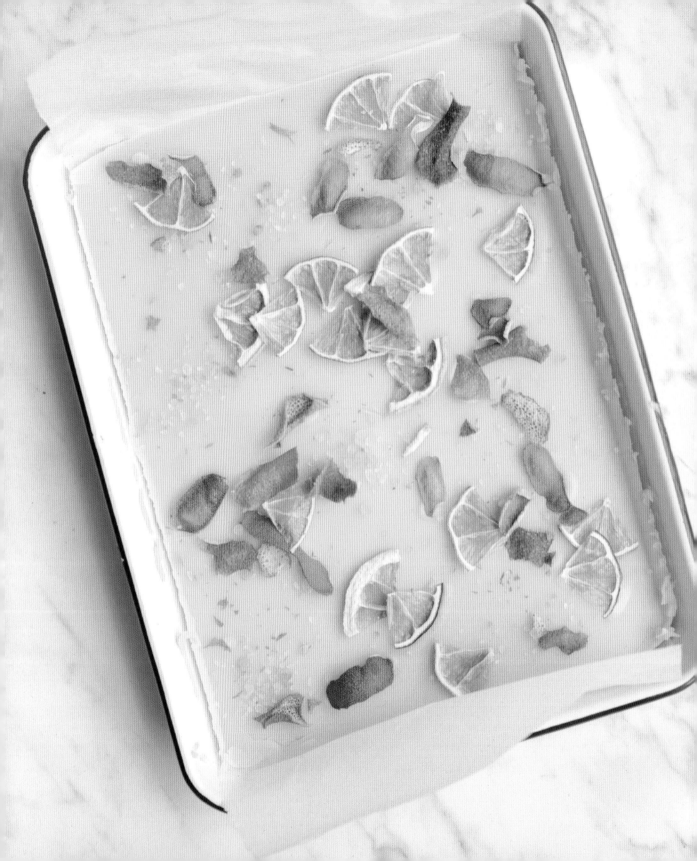

White Chocolate Bath Melt

Like a chocolate bar for your bath, melt this treat into bathwater to create the yummiest experience. The water becomes silky, and the warmth of the water opens the pores and allows the butters and oils to penetrate deeply. You'll emerge from the bath feeling softer than ever! This also happens to be a giftable recipe—a nice treat for the bath lover in your life!

Skin type: all skin types | ***Shelf life:*** 3 months

---

1 cup (218 g) cocoa butter, grated, divided

4 tbsp (60 ml) jojoba oil

40 drops steam-distilled lime essential oil, or your favorite essential oil

Freeze-dried fruit, powdered in a blender, optional (see Tips)

Dried citrus slices, dehydrated in the oven or dehydrator

Dried herbs, dried flowers or dehydrated food, optional

TIPS: If you don't have a bath, make a foot bath version with refreshing peppermint, lemon and lavender essential oils.

If you want to add freeze-dried fruit for color and scent, I recommend that you add it to the oil. Process freeze-dried fruit in a small blender, bullet blender or spice grinder until it forms a fine powder. Pour the jojoba oil into the blender, then blitz again. If there are bits of fruit or seeds in the oil, you can strain them out using a fine-mesh strainer or piece of cheesecloth.

Line a small, shallow baking tray with parchment paper. The ideal size of the tray should be about the size of a chocolate bar, or approximately 5½ inches (14 cm) long by 2½ inches (6 cm) wide. If you don't have a small enough tray, line a food storage container of about that size with parchment paper. You can use a slightly larger size, but if the tray or container is too big, your bar will be thin and melt more quickly in the bath. You want the bath melt to be about ½ inch (1 cm) thick. You can also use chocolate-making molds, found in most craft stores.

Over medium heat, bring a small saucepan of water to a simmer. Set a heatproof bowl over the pot and add half the cocoa butter, stirring continuously for 5 minutes. Then add the remaining cocoa butter, stirring continuously for another 5 minutes over the gently simmering water. It's important to stir continuously, not just to melt the butter, but also to agitate the cocoa butter crystals, so that they will reharden smoothly. Add the jojoba oil.

Remove the bowl from the heat, then add the essential oil and powdered freeze-dried fruit (if using), and stir to incorporate. If this congeals the butter, continue stirring for a minute or two until all the ingredients are fully melted and combined. Working quickly, before the cocoa butter rehardens, pour the mixture onto the parchment paper–lined baking tray.

Set the tray in the freezer for 5 to 10 minutes, until the mixture hardens slightly. Then remove it from the freezer and lightly press in the dried citrus slices and optional dried herbs and flowers, so that they stay at the top and do not sink into the bar.

Let the tray sit on the counter overnight. When the mixture is fully hardened, pop it out and break into pieces. Store in an airtight container.

To use, simply place a bath melt in your bath and let the warm bathwater melt the cocoa butter all over your body! The tub may become a little slippery, so make sure to come out carefully.

SOS Bath Salt

This is a mustard bath, which is an age-old remedy for sore, tired muscles, bodies and minds. Mustard powder is hot; it does not sting, but it does warm up and loosen your muscles. Combined with ginger powder, this bath salt melts tension away. A few drops of cooling peppermint give that hot and cool sensation that seems to work wonders for aching muscles. Try this soak after a workout, or when you've been feeling physically tired, sick or overwhelmed. Mustard also has detoxifying benefits. It's a great way to restore, recover from a hangover and rejuvenate the body.

Skin type: all skin types | ***Shelf life:*** 6 months

---

1 cup (400 g) Epsom salt

1 cup (250 g) magnesium salt

1 tsp jojoba oil

10 drops peppermint essential oil

10 drops lavender essential oil

½ cup (50 g) mustard powder

2 tbsp (10 g) ginger powder

Pour the Epsom and magnesium salts into a large bowl. I love the mix of Epsom and magnesium salts, but you can use all Epsom salt if that's more available to you. In a small bowl, combine the jojoba oil with the peppermint and lavender essential oils, then pour the oil mixture over the salts. Mix well to combine.

In a small bowl, combine the mustard powder and ginger powder, then add them to the salt blend. Mix well. Store in an airtight jar.

To use, add ½ to 1 cup (150 to 300 g) of the bath salt to a bath of warm water to dissolve. Soak for 20 minutes and feel your entire body begin to warm up and relax. I always like to have a drink when bathing. To enhance the effects of this bath from the inside out, make yourself a lemon and ginger tea, and drink it warm or iced.

TIP: You can find mustard powder in the spice aisle of your supermarket. You can make your own ginger powder, dehydrating thinly sliced fresh ginger in the oven at the lowest setting— it will be more fragrant and potent than store bought.

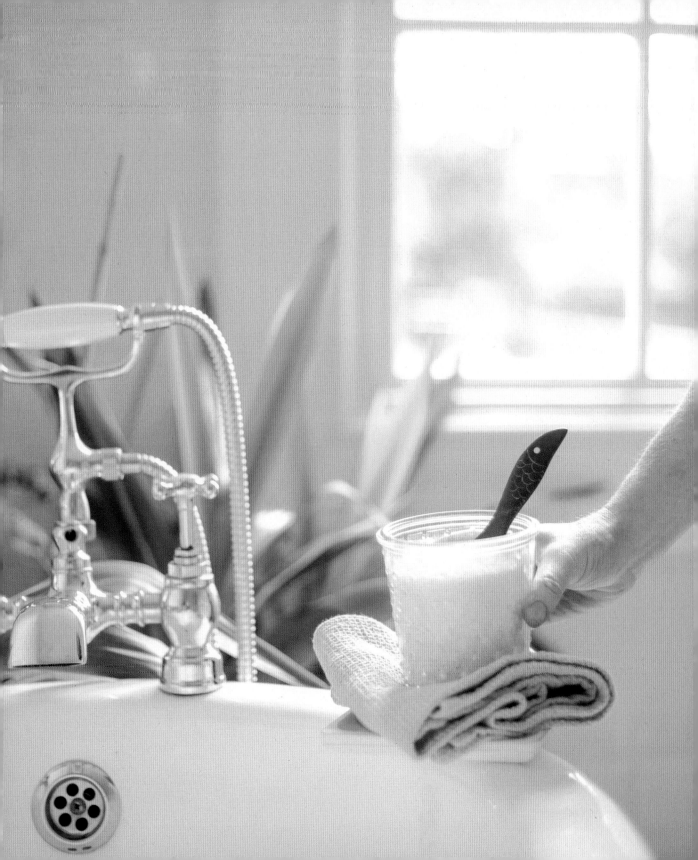

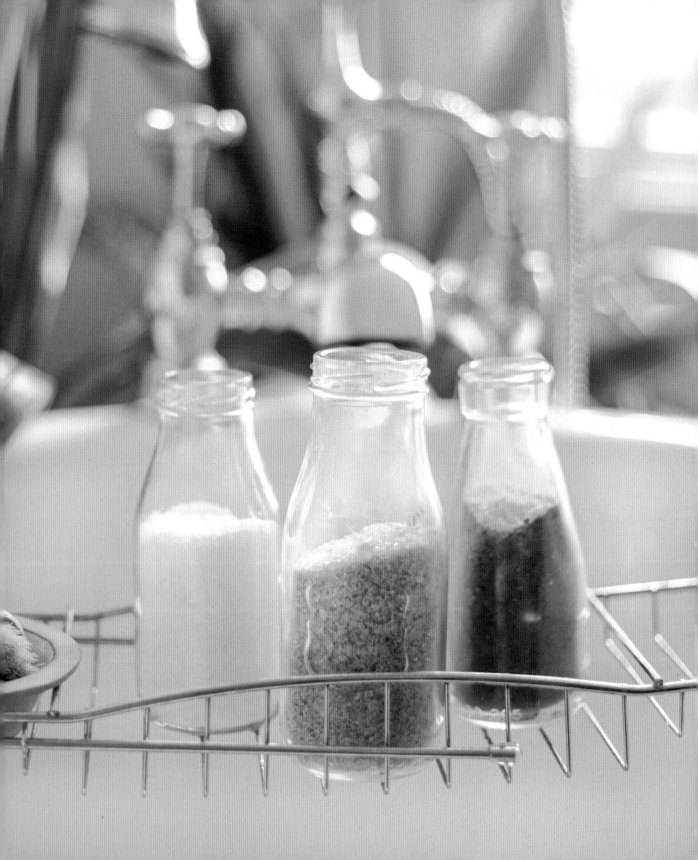

Mylk Bath

Imagine a bathtub of creamy, skin-softening, fragrant mylk. It feels indulgent, but it can be an everyday experience for you. For this recipe, I like using coconut milk because it's moisturizing and smells delicious. You can add in "flavors" of cocoa powder or matcha powder; not only do they create a colorful and fragrant bath but also deliver a ton of antioxidants for your skin to soak up.

Skin type: all skin types | ***Shelf life:*** 3–6 months

---

2 cups (800 g) Epsom salt

½ cup (64 g) coconut milk powder

¼ cup (32 g) matcha powder (see Information about Ingredients, pages 147–148) or cocoa powder, optional

Put the Epsom salts in a blender and process to break down the salt until it reaches a powdery consistency. Add the powdered Epsom salt to a large bowl. Add the coconut milk powder and matcha or cocoa powder (if using). Stir well. Store in an airtight container.

To use, add ½ cup (100 g) to a warm bath. The water will become milky and silky and will feel so incredible on the skin. Soak for 20 minutes in the moisturizing water. I think it's fun to bring a little treat to the bath: a piece of chocolate or a drink to enjoy as you soak!

TIP: If you do not have a bathtub, turn this blend into a body scrub to use in the shower! Epsom salt is too grainy for the skin, so make sure to blitz the salt in a blender to break it down into a finer texture. Add drops of coconut oil and mix until it achieves a wet-sand consistency.

Bath Tea

This bath treat is like a giant cup of tea, giving your skin just what it needs. Chamomile tea calms inflammation, lavender cools redness, calendula stimulates healing and oats soothe and soften. Herbs like rose also have aromatic benefits, soothing nerves and elevating your mood.

Skin type: all skin types | **Shelf life:** 1–3 months

¼ cup (32 g) oat powder (see Information about Ingredients, pages 147–148)

¼ cup (6 g) dried calendula flowers

¼ cup (9 g) dried rose petals

¼ cup (9 g) dried lavender flowers

¼ cup (9 g) dried chamomile flowers

15 drops lavender essential oil

1 tbsp (9 g) grated cocoa butter, optional

Add the oat powder, calendula flowers, rose petals, lavender flowers and chamomile flowers to a small blender, bullet blender or spice grinder. Blitz the ingredients a few times, just to slightly break up the herbs. Pour the blend into an airtight container with a lid, like a Mason jar. Add the lavender essential oil to the mixture along with the grated cocoa butter, if using (this gives the bath a nice creaminess). Close the lid and shake well to incorporate. Store the herbal oat blend in a glass Mason jar by your bath or under the bathroom sink—don't forget to label and date the jar!

To use, scoop out ½ cup (30 g) of Bath Tea into a muslin bag, or tie the mixture into a piece of cheesecloth (this way the herbs will not float off into the bathwater and you can avoid a messy cleanup after your bath!). Add the Bath Tea to the tub as you fill it up, so that it can begin to infuse the water. As you soak, squeeze the bag to release the creamy oat milk; I love splashing it onto my skin and face!

TIP: You can also brew Bath Tea in the kitchen and then pour the herbal tea directly into the bathwater. In a quart-sized (950-ml) Mason jar, add 2 tablespoons each of rolled oats (not oat powder), calendula, rose, lavender and chamomile. Pour 4 cups (960 ml) of hot water from a kettle over the dry ingredients, then close the lid and allow the tea to infuse for 20 minutes. Then strain the liquid through a fine-mesh strainer, and pour directly into the bath. If you wish to add essential oils, combine 1 teaspoon of jojoba oil with 5 drops of essential oil, and pour the oil mixture into the bath.

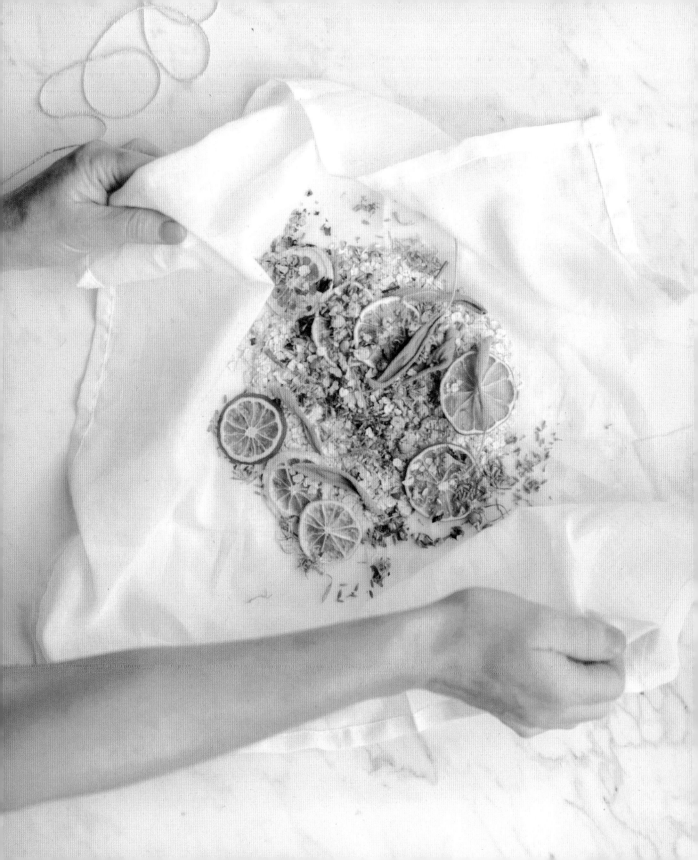

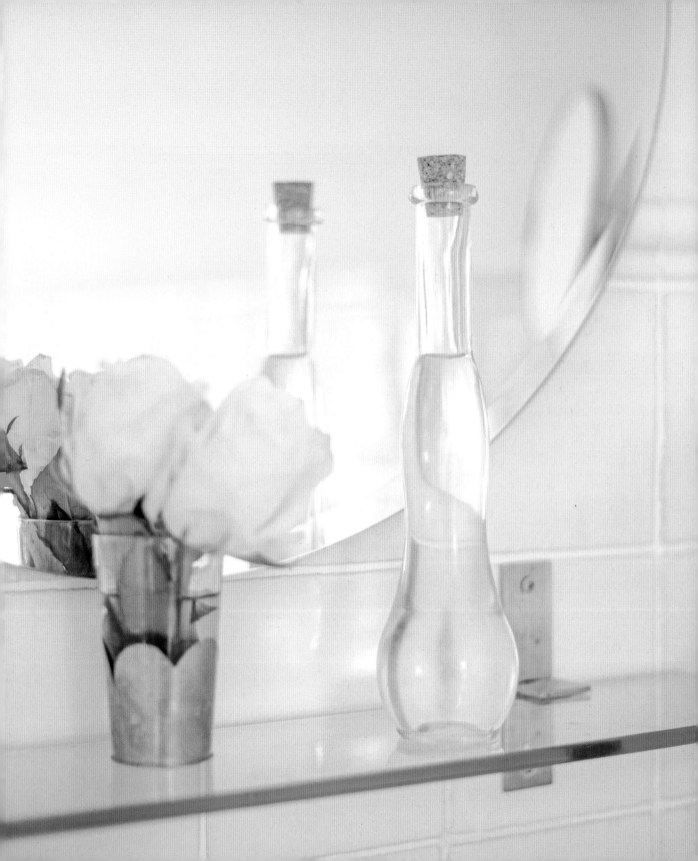

Body Splash

A body splash is a light perfume, perfect for any time of the day, but I think it's especially nice before slipping into bed. My mom used to use Agua de Florida every night after her shower, and I loved watching her splash her neck and shoulders. Now any time that I come across that scent, it sends me right back to those happy memories. I love the idea of creating a signature scent and using it intentionally during a time in life you want to preserve. Scent and emotion are connected and create strong memories, so any time you smell that same aroma, you're instantly transported to that time and the way you felt.

This recipe is inspired by my childhood memories, with essential oils creating the fragrance. It may be your new scent—or the inspiration to create your own special blend.

Skin type: all skin types | *Shelf life:* 3–6 months

---

1 cup (240 ml) witch hazel

¼ cup (9 g) dried rose petals

¼ cup (9 g) dried lavender flowers

1 cinnamon stick, or 2 drops cinnamon essential oil

15 drops rose geranium essential oil

3 drops lemon essential oil

3 drops lavender essential oil

3 drops orange essential oil

In a Mason jar, combine the witch hazel with the rose petals, lavender and cinnamon stick (if using). Seal the lid and let the mixture sit for 1 day, then strain out the solids and return the infused witch hazel to the jar.

Add the rose geranium, cinnamon (if using), lemon, lavender and orange essential oils to the witch hazel, and swirl or stir to combine.

You can keep this mixture in a spray bottle, but if you also like the idea of splashing your skin after a shower, bottle it in a container from which you can pour the splash into your hand. Shake before use to distribute the oils.

To use, splash liberally all over—neck, chest and body.

TIP: Although it takes time, infusing herbs gives a wonderful aroma and you get the extra benefit of the healing constituents from the plants. Traditionally an infusion sits for weeks to extract out the medicinal components of a plant; but for the aroma, one day will do the job. If you don't want to infuse the witch hazel with dried herbs, you can skip it and add only essential oils to create your fragrance.

Personal Space Mist

No matter where you are, create a space around you that makes you feel fresh, uplifted and clean. I love having this on hand when I'm out to spray on my clothes or my hands to disinfect. You can spray the bathroom or the air around you. Like a smokeless sage cleansing stick, it's great to spray the air in your car or home to clear away stale odors—to make you feel more relaxed, safe and happy. Sage is one of my favorite essential oils—it lifts mental fatigue and lethargy, lightens a heavy mood and focuses the mind. In folk herbalism, it was thought to promote increased wisdom, like the "wise sage."

Skin type: all skin types | *Shelf life:* 3–6 months

---

1 oz (30 ml) 90–100% ethanol (such as grain alcohol)

25 drops sage essential oil

10 drops lavender essential oil

20 drops lemon essential oil

3 oz (90 ml) purified water

Add the alcohol to a 4-ounce (120-ml) glass spray bottle, then add the sage, lavender and lemon essential oils. Fill the bottle with the purified water.

To use, shake first and then spray all over your clothes, the air and furniture.

TIPS: You can increase the essential oils, up to double the amount listed in the recipe. Start with this smaller amount, and build up if you prefer a stronger scent.

Alternative purifying oils you can try include thyme, tea tree, lemongrass, rosemary, eucalyptus and hyssop. You can use witch hazel instead of alcohol, but the benefit of using such a high-proof alcohol is that it both preserves the product and also helps to disperse the essential oils.

Make yourself a travel-size container for on-the-go use.

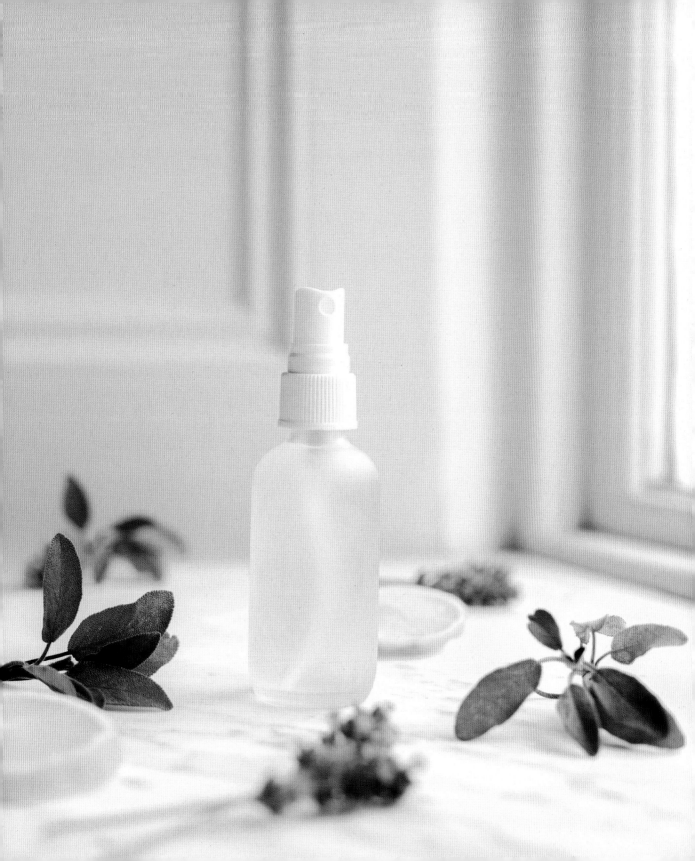

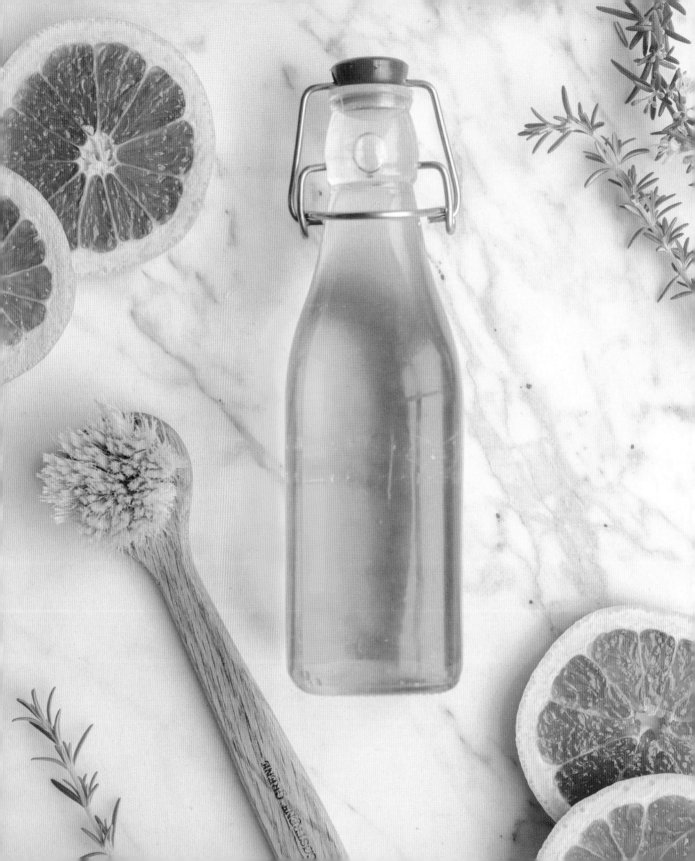

Clarifying Hair Rinse

Vinegar is one of the best hair-care ingredients; it helps to remove product buildup, stimulates the scalp, clears hair follicles and leaves your hair smooth and glossy. Unlike oil treatments or products, a hair rinse does not coat and weigh down the hair—it rinses completely clean. I know people who have successfully cut out the shampoo, using hair rinse as a cleanser and conditioner! Start small, and use this hair rinse once per week as a "clarifying treatment." You'll be surprised how effective this remedy can be! For this recipe, we're infusing vinegar with fragrant, stimulating herbs to promote healthy hair growth.

Skin type: all skin types | **Shelf life:** 3–6 months

¼ cup (7 g) dried or fresh rosemary

¼ cup (7 g) dried or fresh lavender flowers (if using fresh, you can also use the leaves of the plant)

3–4 cups (0.75–1 L) apple cider vinegar

Fill a large, clean jar with the dried herbs, and top it off with the apple cider vinegar, to about 1 inch (3 cm) above the herbs. Let the mixture sit to infuse for at least 2 weeks and up to 4 weeks. Shake the jar every couple of days to encourage the constituents out of the herbs. When you are ready to use, strain out the herbs and pour the herbal vinegar into a glass bottle. This is your stock; you will take some from this for each treatment.

To use, fill a squeeze bottle (an empty condiment bottle or hair dye application bottle) one quarter of the way with the infused herbal vinegar, then fill the rest with water. In the shower, wet your hair or shampoo as normal. Then apply the tip of the bottle to your scalp and begin to squeeze out the Clarifying Hair Rinse all over your scalp. Gather your hair and saturate it with the rinse. Massage your head, making sure the product is all over your scalp, then rinse clean under the stream of water.

If you feel like you need it, you can add a little conditioner to the tips of your hair. But try using just the hair rinse and see how your hair responds to it without added products.

TIP: You can use essential oils instead of infusing if you prefer. Add 20 drops of essential oil per 1 cup (240 ml) of apple cider vinegar.

Edible Body Oil

This oil is simply delicious; your skin will smell and taste like a chocolate dessert. Apply it all over your body—it can be used head to toe. The ingredients are completely edible. You can use Edible Body Oil as a lubricant and for genital massage, but for safe play, do not use this oil with latex condoms because the coconut oil can cause breakage. This oil is beautiful to wear any time of day as a fragrance. Vanilla is an aphrodisiac and elevates the mood; it's warming and lingers on the skin.

Skin type: all skin types | **Shelf life:** 3–6 months

---

1 oz (30 ml) melted coconut oil

1 oz (30 ml) jojoba oil

2 tsp (5 g) cacao nibs (see Tips)

½ vanilla bean pod (see Tips)

Use the warm method to infuse the coconut and jojoba oils with the cacao nibs and vanilla pod in just 6 hours (see Herbal-Infused Oil 101 on pages 18–19).

When the oil is infused, strain out the cacao nibs and the vanilla pod and reserve the fragrant oil in a bottle of your choice. To use, massage onto your skin.

TIPS: Cacao nibs are broken-down pieces of cacao (or cocoa) beans; they have a chocolaty aroma and flavor. You can find them in most supermarkets and health-food stores.

I always slice open a vanilla bean pod and scrape out the inner seeds to use in my baking and use just the pods to infuse oil for my skin care. You can also add the seeds to a jar of sugar; you can then use this vanilla sugar for baking.

Pour this blend into a bath, or use it to make Body Butter (page 80) or Solid Body Moisturizer (page 64).

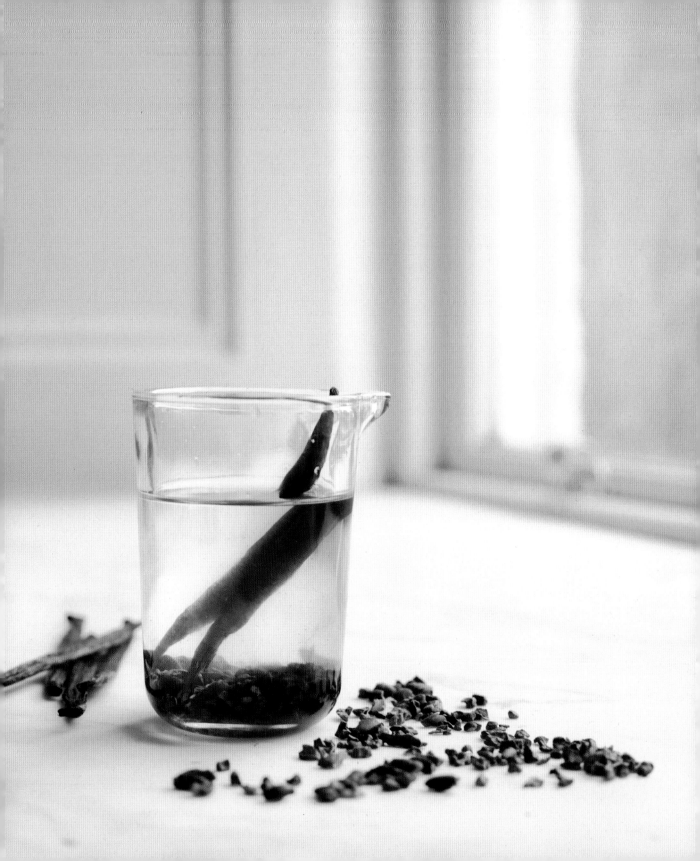

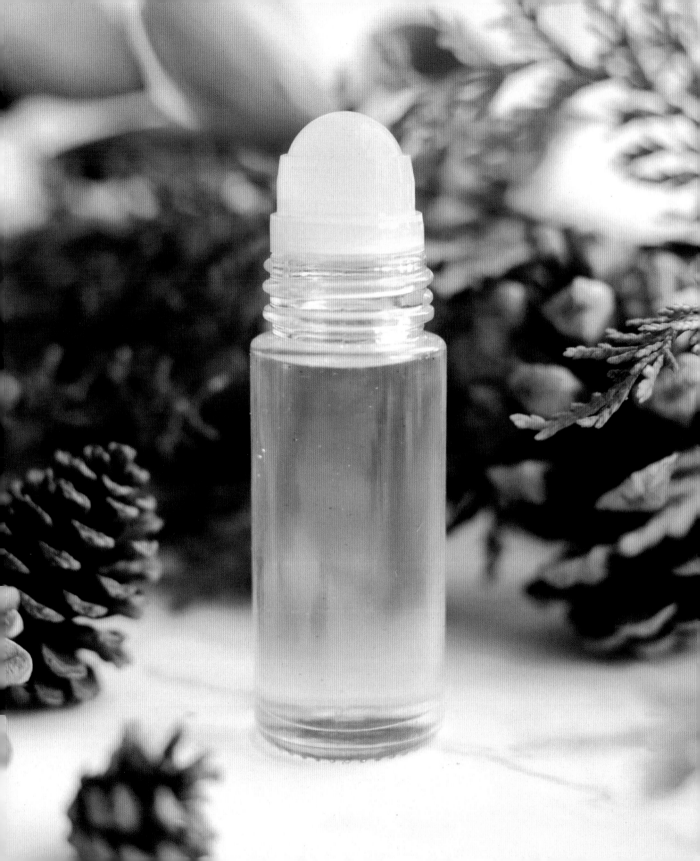

Forest Bathing Body Mist

I love traveling to forested areas with my family, I always feel completely restored in the clear air, and I wanted to capture that feeling in this recipe. Studies have looked at the effects of being surrounded by nature, finding that just being in a green forest environment reduces stress levels and restores the mind and body. Forest bathing has become a popular wellness exercise, people walking among the trees to change the way they feel. I wish I had a forest in my backyard, but for everyday de-stressing, this spray will make you feel like you're there!

Skin type: all skin types | **Shelf life:** 6 months

Body & Room Spray

1 oz (30 ml) 90–100% ethanol (such as grain alcohol)

25 drops white fir essential oil

18 drops spruce essential oil

7 drops peppermint essential oil

3 oz (90 ml) purified water

Rollerball

2 tsp (10 ml) jojoba oil

5 drops white fir essential oil

3 drops spruce essential oil

2 drops peppermint oil

To make the spray version, add the alcohol to a glass spray bottle, then drop in the white fir, spruce and peppermint essential oils. Swirl to mix, then add the water.

To use, spray into the room, breathe in the air and feel yourself relax.

To make the rollerball version (see Tips), add the jojoba oil to the rollerball. Add the white fir, spruce and peppermint essential oils.

To use, roll it over your hands, and then cusp your hands over your nose and breathe deeply. Apply to your neck and wrists to keep the scent with you.

TIPS: The rollerball recipe will fit in a 10-milliliter rollerball; you can find rollerball applicators online or in craft-supply stores.

You can use alternative essential oils that offer the same forest bathing effect: atlas cedarwood, cypress, pine or Douglas fir. You can use any blend of oils you would like in whatever combination; any combination should total 50 drops for the spray version and 10 drops for the rollerball version.

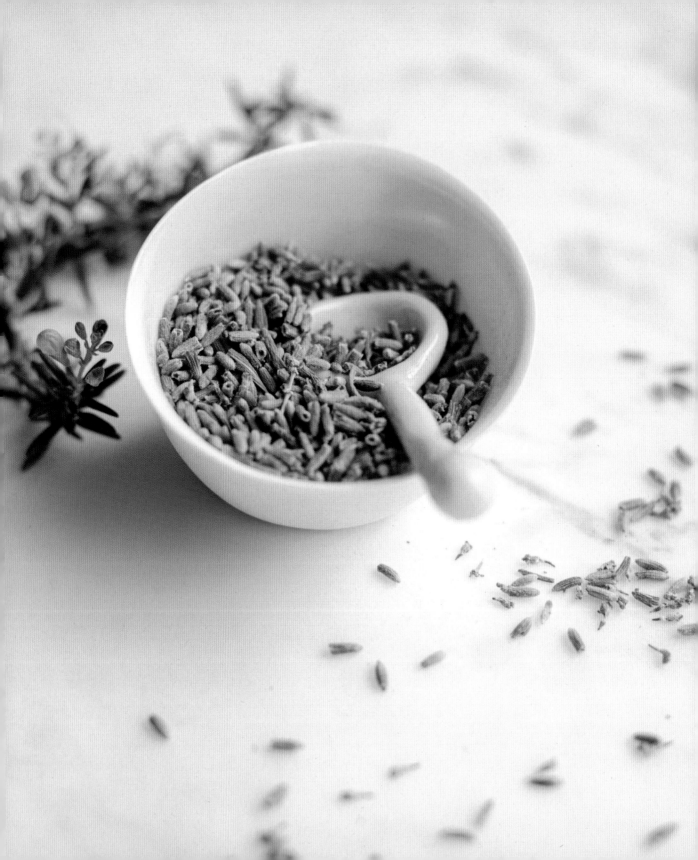

Information about Ingredients

Dried Herbs

You can find dried herbs, like chamomile and lavender, in the tea section of your local supermarket. Look for brands that focus on quality herbs and use no colorings or flavorings. Check if your area has an herb store where you can purchase a wide variety of herbs. Or you can purchase herbs online. My favorite suppliers include:

Mountain Rose Herbs: https://www.mountainroseherbs.com/

Starwest Botanicals: https://www.starwest-botanicals.com/

Frontier Co-Op: https://www.frontiercoop.com/

My journey into making skin-care products began in Singapore. For my Singaporean community, I recommend:

Abundant Earth: https://www.abundantearth.sg/

Herbal Powders

Many of the recipes, like the masks and scrubs, call for an herbal powder (for example, rose powder, oat powder, calendula powder, lavender powder and so on). You can purchase herbal powders online; I recommend:

Mountain Rose Herbs: https://www.mountainroseherbs.com

However, you can also make these powders yourself at home, simply by grinding the whole herb or ingredient in a small blender, bullet blender or coffee grinder. I recommend blitzing approximately 1 cup (240 g) of the ingredient until it becomes powdery fine. Store your homemade herbal powder in a labeled jar in the pantry. You can then use it for other recipes as needed. Herbal powders last for about 6 months in the pantry.

Freeze-Dried Fruit and Fruit Powders

You can find freeze-dried fruit in the snack section of health-food stores and many supermarkets. In any recipe that calls for freeze-dried fruit, you can use fresh fruit if you prefer! It will lower the shelf life of your product to 1 to 3 days, but that just means your face masks will be totally fresh!

Some recipes call for freeze-dried fruit powders. To make the powder yourself, simply blitz the freeze-dried fruit pieces in a small blender, bullet blender or coffee grinder. I recommend storing fruit powder in the freezer where it will stay powdery and bone dry.

Orange Peel Powder

You can make your own orange peel powder by dehydrating an orange peel in the oven and then powdering it in a blender. It's a great way to use up the peel, rather than throwing it away! Set your oven to its lowest setting, and place the orange peels on a parchment paper–covered baking tray. Set the tray in the oven for 20 to 30 minutes, checking the peel periodically. I prefer to leave the oven door slightly cracked during this process so the oven doesn't get too hot. For more complete instructions, search for "How to Make a Batch of Dried Orange Peel" on my website at https://littlegreendot.com/. After the peels are dried, blitz them in a small blender, bullet blender or coffee grinder. I recommend storing the orange peel powder in a labeled jar in the pantry. It will keep for up to 6 months.

Clay Powders

Most health-food stores sell bentonite clay in the beauty section, often under the name "Indian healing clay." This can be used for any recipe in the book calling for clay. Bentonite clay is a "thirstier" clay, and you may find that you need to add more water than called for in the recipes. I recommend kaolin clay for drier skin types, as it is very gentle. For kaolin clay and other varieties of clay, I recommend:

Mountain Rose Herbs: https://www.mountainroseherbs.com/

From Nature With Love: https://www.fromnaturewithlove.com/

Coconut Milk Powder, Milk Powders and Colloidal Oats

For some of the more "specialty" ingredients, plus oils, butters, clays and more, I recommend:

From Nature with Love: https://www.fromnaturewithlove.com/

Oils

You can find wonderful oils for your skin-care needs in the supermarket. You'll easily find avocado, almond, coconut oil and more; I suggest that you look on the very top and lower bottom shelves for the better selection of unrefined oils.

For jojoba oil specifically (which I love for all skin types), I recommend:

The Jojoba Company: https://www.jojobacompany.com/

For more specialty oils—for example, rosehip seed or argan oil to make the Facial Serum (page 71)— I recommend:

Lotus Garden Botanicals: https://www.lgbotanicals.com/

Butters

Some health-food stores sell shea butter. You'll find cocoa butter in the baking section of the supermarket. To purchase online, I recommend:

Better Shea Butter & Skin Foods: https://bettersheabutter.com/

Also, if you love experimenting and want to create something unique, you can find a larger variety of butters on the websites From Nature With Love and Lotus Garden Botanicals.

Essential Oils

It's "essential" that you purchase your essential oils from a reputable brand that focuses on purity, quality and sustainability. I recommend the following suppliers:

Mountain Rose Herbs: https://www.mountainroseherbs.com/

Plant Therapy: https://www.planttherapy.com/

Aura Cacia: https://www.auracacia.com

Floracopeia: https://www.floracopeia.com/

Lotus Garden Botanicals: https://www.lgbotanicals.com/

Flavor Oils

For the lip balm and lip scrubs, you can use any brand of flavoring found in your supermarket, but I recommend using real candy flavoring:

LorAnn Oils: https://www.lorannoils.com/

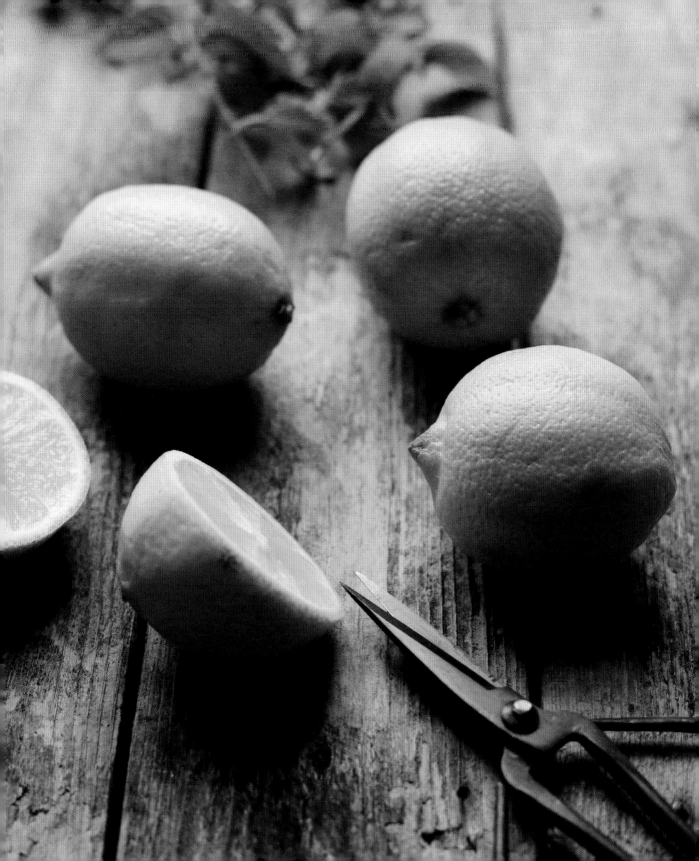

Acknowledgments

I want to thank my husband, Ciaran—you encouraged me every step of the way, back when I decided to dedicate myself to learning herbal skin care, even though I had no idea where it was all leading. Dad, you showed me how using curiosity and creativity can create better solutions. Mom, you showed me the importance of community and of being of service to others.

I feel really lucky to have had an amazing team by my side: Page Street Publishing. Thank you so much for helping me along the process of writing my first book!

I shot the photos for the book in Ireland, with a talented food stylist named Karen Colvery. When I called her to ask her to work on this skin-care book, she said, "Well, I actually work with food. . . . " and I said, "So do I!" Thank you so much, Karen, for seeing the vision and helping me to translate food as skin care! Brendan and Josie, thank you for giving me a home in Ireland, full of good food and good energy, so that I could create this work. It made all the difference!

I've had many mentors who sparked my curiosity and interest in herbalism. John Gallagher, Rosemary Gladstar, Susun Weed, John Green—I especially appreciate, beyond the information that you teach, the deep reverence for nature you instill in all who learn from you.

Thank you to my herbal school, Florida School of Holistic Living—you opened me up to a community of herbalist friends, the best teachers and hands-on learning that I could have ever wanted!

And I have to thank *you*, the person reading this book! Even if you don't know it, you gave me such a strong sense of purpose, to create the best recipes I could and to learn every day, so that I could share it with you.

About the Author

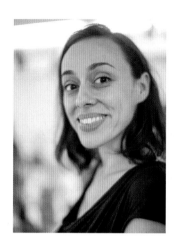

Militza Maury moved back to Florida in 2017, where she now lives with her husband, two daughters and their dog, Bali. Her journey into skin care and herbalism began in Singapore, where she lived for 15 years. There in her tiny kitchen, she learned how to make skin-care products for her own family, as a home herbalist. She then studied formally, becoming a community herbalist to support clients on their health journey. Militza also spent two years with her family living in Bali, where she learned from traditional skin-care makers, outside in the open air. Her passion for nature and food have come together in the form of natural whole food skin care that she teaches in workshops and online. On most days, you'll find her in her kitchen, dehydrating slices of lemons or infusing herbs in jars, developing new recipes and sharing her creations on her website, Little Green Dot.

Index